HYGGE

HAPPINESS NOW

Danish Secrets, How to Be Happy with a Simple Lifestyle

LARS JOHANSEN

TABLE OF CONTENTS

Chapter # 2

Chapter # 3

Chapter # 6

How to Practice Hygge for Winter Self-care 110

CHAPTER # 1

Hygge Happiness Now

The new World Happiness Report again positions Denmark among the best three happiest of 155 countries reviewed—a distinction that the country has earned for seven consecutive years.

The US, then again, ranked eighteenth right now Happiness Report, a four-spot drop from last year's report.

Denmark's place among the world's happiest countries is reliable with numerous other national surveys of happiness (or, as psychologists call it, "subjective health").

Researchers like to study and argue about how to measure things. In any case, with regards to satisfaction, a consensus appears to have developed.

Depending upon the scope and reason for the research, happiness is regularly estimated utilizing objective indicators (information on crime, pay, metro commitment, and health) and subjective techniques, for example, asking people how as often as possible they experience positive and negative feelings.

For what reason may Danes assess their lives all the more positively? As an analyst and local of Denmark, I've looked into this question.

Indeed, Danes have a steady government, low degrees of public corruption, and high-quality education and health care. The nation has the most elevated assessments in the world; however, by far, most of Danes happily pay: They accept higher taxes can make a better society.

Maybe in particular, however, they esteem a social development called "hygge" (articulated hʊgə).

The Oxford dictionary included the word in June 2017, and it refers to great social associations. Hygge can be utilized as a thing, descriptive word or verb (to hygge oneself), and occasions and places can also be hyggelige (hygge-like).

Hygge is some of the time translated as "cozy," however a superior meaning of hygge is "intentional intimacy," which can happen when you have safe, adjusted, and agreeable shared experiences. Some coffee with a friend before a chimney may qualify, as could a summer picnic in the park.

A family may have a hygge evening that involves table games and treats, or friends may get together for a casual dinner with diminished lighting, great nourishment, and easygoing fun. Spaces can also be described as hyggelige ("Your new house is so hyggeligt"), and a typical method for telling a host thank you after a dinner is to state that it was hyggeligt (which means, we made some great memories). Most Danish get-togethers are required to be hyggelige, so it would be a harsh critique to state that a party or dinner wasn't hyggelige.

Research on hygge has discovered that in Denmark, it's integral to people's feeling of health. It goes about as a buffer against stress, while additionally making space to assemble fellowship. In a highly individualized country like Denmark, hygge can advance egalitarianism and strengthen trust.

It is reasonable for the state that hygge is completely coordinated into the Danish social mind and culture. But, it has additionally gotten somewhat of a worldwide phenomenon—Amazon currently sells more than 900 books on hygge, and Instagram has more than 3 million posts with the hashtag #hygge. Google trends information show a major jump in searches for hygge starting in October 2016.

Nor is Denmark the only country that has a word for an idea like hygge—the Norwegians have koselig, the Swedes mysig, the Dutch gezenlligheid, and the Germans gemütlichkeit.

In the US—which additionally puts a high value on individualism—there's no genuine social likeness hygge. Salary is by and large connected with happiness, yet although the nation's GDP has been increasing, and its unemployment rates have been declining, levels of happiness in the US have been consistently reducing.

What's happening?

Income inequality keeps on being an issue. But at the same time, there's been a marked decrease in relational trust and trust toward establishments like the government just as the media. At last, more disposable income doesn't measure up to having somebody to depend on in a time of need (something that 95% of Danes accept they have).

At its center, hygge is tied in with building closeness and trust with others.

Americans could most likely utilize somewhat more of it in their lives.

Hygge: Unlocking Denmark's Secret to Happiness

In the relatively recent past, Americans' information on Denmark pretty much began with Hamlet and finished with an unpopular cheese-filled pastry.

That has changed since Demark turned into a worldwide leader with the nourishment wonder Noma, its binge-worthy crime dramas "The Killing" and "Borgen," and a structured sense that has everybody desiring light wood and sheepskins.

So it wouldn't have been long until Americans began wondering about another Danish marvel: One of the happiest populations on the planet, as indicated by yearly reviews by the United Nations, among others.

Enter hygge (articulated "hoo-ga"). It's a Danish word without an exact simple, however, approximately interpreted as comfortable satisfaction. It's a significant piece of the Danish world view — individuals talk about how hyggeligt it will be to get together, and how hyggelig that social affair was. Also, it's the subject of a way of life publishing boom.

Fitting to Denmark's atmosphere (and our winter), hygge is tied in with digging in's: everything candles, blazing flames, warm covers, and fuzzy slippers, reading books (called hyggekrog), comfort jeans (hyggebukser), wollen socks (hyggesokker) and tea.

Hygge in Denmark

I experienced childhood in Denmark, and I moved to the United States when I was 18 years of age. Having lived for a long time in the two societies has given me the extraordinary knowledge to take the best from both worlds – and an incredible piece of that is incorporating Danish hygge into American life.

Denmark was an amazing spot to grow up. I genuinely had the happiest childhood. I was parented "the Danish Way" and was an awesome spot to bring up your youngsters. Anyway, this probably won't be a possibility for everybody. Hygge is an approach to bring the Danish way of life and Danish satisfaction into your own home! One of the manners in which you can raise happy and certain kids is by practicing hygge as a family and incorporating it into your home and everyday lifestyle.

The basic craft of feeling content, happy, and comfortable

Sometime before I knew about the Danish word hygge (articulated practically like "hyuu-guh"), and before hygge turned into a worldwide pattern, I was longing forever delights that energized a feeling of happiness and health. Nothing on a grand scale, mind you— simply the seemingly insignificant details that cause you to feel warm and fuzzy inside. Slipping on a couple of cloud-delicate aloe-implanted socks on a cool night, lighting a flame in the kitchen window on an overcast morning, or decorating my breakfast nook with a simple vase of wildflowers. Furthermore, that pot of Provençal stew gradually braising in the broiler on a winter's day, with the expectation of dinner close to a crackling fire—perfection. Much to my dismay, I was looking for hygge.

The Good Life, Hygge Style

All in all, what precisely is the meaning of hygge? There's no equivalent English word, although comfort approaches. Hygge is tied in with discovering basic things that carry comfort and satisfaction to your body and soul and then appreciating those experiences. Take candlelight—something pretty much everybody agrees is super hygge. Lighting a wick until you have a fire isn't hygge all by itself. Candles become hygge when you easily revel in their comfy glowing light. You feel this from inside, and it's deeply calming. Well, that is, hygge!

Is hygge a sort of care, also—another trendy expression

that has caught our consideration of late? While hygge and care are not fundamentally unrelated, I think "presence" is more proper than "care." Mindful methods being attentive and aware; however, it can also mean being careful. It doesn't appear that hygge includes conscious carefulness. Rather, it's the sheer simplicity of experiencing comfort and then enclosing yourself by that feeling without forcing it.

Maybe it's simpler to describe what hygge doesn't involve—materialism, gluttony, envy, and excess. Having a colossal house, driving the fastest car on the block, or conveying the most recent designer handbag (as a matter of fact, one of my guilty pleasures) aren't hygge. It isn't around one-increasing your neighbors or hanging out online either, because, in a hygge world, direct social collaboration, individual warmth, and genuine nature are valued.

WHAT DOES HYGGE MEAN?

The feeling of hygge runs somewhere down in Danish culture. Denmark is reliably positioned as perhaps the happiest countries in the world – for 2019, it earned the No. 2 spot in the World Happiness Report, simply behind Finland.

Hygge, at its center, is a feeling. It tends to be

welcomed by getting a charge out of the simple pleasures of life, similar to a warm drink on a stormy day or time that went through relaxing with friends.

Hygge isn't a way of life pattern that expects you to purchase lots of new things or go moderate and dispose of all your natural belongings. It's the feeling you get when you're enveloped with a soft blanket with a candle flickering on the table alongside you. Anybody can practice hygge as they are at present.

While "hygge" is regularly utilized as a thing or an adjective, it can also be utilized as an action word. For instance, in Danish culture, you can hygge. Something can also be hyggelig (hygge-like), like a restaurant or an event.

10 ELEMENTS OF HYGGE

As per "The Little Book of Hygge," there are 10 components in The Hygge Manifesto. You needn't bother with each of these to experience hygge, yet the more you have, the more hyggelig the circumstance or condition is. The components are as per the following:

Air

A hygge-like air has low, soft lighting. This is

frequently achieved with bunches of candles.

Nearness

There's an emphasis in hygge on being completely present while spending time with your friends and family. No telephones, no PCs, no interruptions.

Pleasure

Hygge is tied in with getting a charge out of simple pleasures, as hot drinks, cakes, treats, and other sweet treats.

Equality

A hygge-like social event ensures nobody individual takes on a lot of the talking or the responsibility for tasks. Everybody finds a good pace; everybody causes each other – it's "we" over "me."

Gratitude

The individuals who practice hygge place center around appropriately taking in every basic minute and valuing it for what it is.

Amicability

Hygge urges people to remember that they aren't in

rivalry with their friends and family and shouldn't want to boast about their achievements to acquire a greater amount of their warmth. At a hygge-like social event, things flow peacefully

Comfort

To achieve hygge, you must be comfortable. Agreeable garments and furniture and a comfortable, relaxing condition are significant.

Truce

At a hygge-like occasion, you don't discuss disruptive themes like governmental issues. Table any arguments or sources of pressure and appreciate the time you're going through with your friends and family.

Togetherness

Hygge should be possible alone, yet it's best in little groups. At hygge-like events, time ought to be spent structure and strengthening your associations with individuals whose company you enjoy.

Shelter

Eventually, past the environment and the treats, hygge is tied in with having a sense of security. You're with individuals you trust in a spot that feels peaceful and secure.

APPROACHES TO ADD HYGGE DECOR IN YOUR HOME

The primary thing to recognize is that hygge can happen anyplace; in any case, it's frequently done in the home. It should also be possible whenever of year, yet figuring in the significance of comfort, winter may be the ideal time for you to begin on your hygge journey. Here are a couple of things you can focus on to make your place more hygge-like.

Get Cozy

Get creative with how you consolidate hygge-like decor layout into your living space during the colder months. Think plush furniture, warm hide or polar fluffy knit accent pillows, and anything else that makes you need to snuggle up before a roaring fire.

The Danes organize comfort such a lot of that having an alcove or a "comfortable corner" is normal.

"The 'hyggekrug,' or comfortable corner, is a foundation of hygge. Making one in the room makes an ideal little hygge oasis," notes Jordan Zaplatosch, public relations specialist with home goods organization LuxeDecor, "Delicate materials, similar to a hide carpet or cover, with lush pillows makes a feeling of relaxation and rejuvenation."

Light the Candles

Candles are a practically vital part of the hygge way of life. According to a study done by the Happiness Research Institute and distributed in "The Little Book of Hygge," over 70% of Danes light candles in any event once per week, and 28% light them consistently. They're not simply lighting one flame, either, as 31% of individuals in Denmark will in general light more than five at once.

Maureen Calamia of Luminous Spaces, a Feng shui counseling and preparing business, says, "The most significant thing in hygge is the lighting. Delicate lighting with candles and lights that emanate warm/yellow lighting."

Pick candles in different shapes and sizes that mix well together. In case you decide on a scented flame, focus on wintry scents that are normal, similar to pine, or ones that are warm and sugary, similar to occasion treats and other baked goods.

Go Natural

Hygge gives close attention to common components. Hygge configuration regularly includes wood and different components that attach the decor back to nature.

"My greatest takeaway from hygge is the standards of authenticity and expectation. Handcrafted objects made of common materials … make a feeling of caring and warmth," says Calamia.

In "The Little Book of Hygge," Wiking refers to that wood is a key factor in a hygge-like home, yet that wood alone isn't sufficient. "Danes want to bring the entire forest inside," written Wiking, "Any bit of nature you may find is probably going to get the hygge green light." To make your hygge winter wonderland, consider layering animal hides (false ones included) with your wooden components and including other snowy characteristic contacts, similar to pine festoons, pinecones, wreaths, berries, and twigs. Possibly sprinkle a touch of fake snow on your racks!

Assemble

Togetherness is one of the key components of hygge, so it should not shock anyone that social occasion is a fast method to hygge. Zaplatosch noticed, "A general feeling of hospitality and warmth are a portion of the key components of this [hygge] style."

Having little groups of individuals over to draw in with is a typical event for some individuals in Denmark. 78% of Danes state they associate in any event once every week, as indicated by "The Little Book of Hygge." This winter, consider welcoming your closest friends and family into your home once in a while to huddle together against the chilly, share some hot drinks and sweet treats, and appreciate each other's company.

Having things in your home that make facilitating simpler is additionally an incredible method to incorporate hygge. Decide on kitchen basics like serving plate, ceramic drinkware, and tables that individuals can easily sit around.

If, in the wake of learning this, you're prepared to get comfortable (and perhaps twist up and sleep), you're prepared for hygge. Winter is an extraordinary time to start your quest for hygge – with this chilly weather, coziness, and warmth may be the jolt of energy you need. But, hygge is something you can make progress toward all year, significantly after the ground starts to thaw.

Definitions of Hygge

Since English has no word for hygge, most stories about the thought begin by attempting to define it. Nation Living depicts it as "a feeling of comfortable satisfaction and health through getting a charge out of the basic things throughout everyday life." British writer Helen Russell, writer of "The Year of Living Danishly," calls it "enjoying the presence of gentle, relieving things." Oxford Living Dictionaries characterizes it as "nature of comfort and agreeable conviviality that engenders a feeling of happiness or well-being."

However, no concise definition truly gets at the core of what hygge means. A superior method to understand it is to take a look at things that individuals describe as hygge and what they share practically speaking. Instances of the hygge life will, in general offer five main features:

- Comfort. In his book, Wiking relates one of his most loved hygge memories. He's going through Christmas Day with a group of friends in a lodge in the woods. After a long climb in the day off, sit together around a log fire, wearing sweaters and fleece socks, sipping mulled wine. The entire scene radiates comfort:

the glow and crackle of the fire, the comfortable sweaters, the hot wine, all set against the chilly, blanketed foundation. The main thing that could make it more hygge, they agree, is to have a storm raging outside.

- Companionship. Something else that makes Wiking's scene so perfectly hygge is the group of friends sharing it. You can do hygge things without anyone else, for example, sitting on the lounge chair with a book, a cover, and some tea, yet it's twice as hygge to share experiences with other people. Little get-togethers are best for this intention; it's a lot cozier to spend time with a couple of dear friends than with a major group of strangers, either in broad daylight or on the Internet. Alex Beauchamp, who online journals at Hygge House, says hygge is regularly described as an "art of creating closeness."

- Relaxation. This isn't a similar thing as sitting still. For example, going for a walk through the forested areas on a fall day, particularly with a group of friends, can be very hygge – however, it must be a relaxed walk. Getting some activity is fine, however any suggestion of haste or rush crown jewels the state of mind. Claus Meyer, a Danish chief, clarifies in the New York Times article that when Danes assemble for dinner, they frequently start with appetizers, at that point, go out for a two-hour walk before the main meal. This unhurried pace is a piece of the hygge experience.

- Connection to Nature. Although it's acceptable to be comfortable inside, a full hygge life includes spending time outside as well. John Crace of the Happiness Research Institute, writing for The Guardian, says Danes even appreciate going out in the rain. Living hygge means getting a charge out of the sights, sounds, and smells of nature: a rainstorm outside the window, honking blaring overhead, flowers in bloom. Cooking with new, common fixings is also part of the hygge way of life; in "How to Hygge," Johansen incorporates plans for New Nordic Cuisine claims to fame, for example, muesli, organic product compote, and roast sheep. You can give your home a hyggelig feel by getting the outside with fresh blossoms or uncovered branches, or by killing the electric lights and lighting a few candles so you can watch the flames. Indeed, even line-drying your clothing, with your perfect towels snapping in the breeze, is an approach to feel hygge (and save money on clothing costs at the same time).

- Simplicity. Hygge is tied in with getting a charge out of the simple things throughout everyday life, not chasing after thrills. Beauchamp says it requires "the capacity to be available – as well as perceive and appreciate the present." Sipping your morning coffee in your shower robe while sitting by an open window – or better despite everything, out on the porch – tuning in to the fowls sing is hygge. Running into Starbucks for a to-go cup on your approach to work, while all the while tuning in to music and checking Facebook on your telephone, isn't.

Examples of Hygge

Articles about hygge will, in general, focus on wintertime exercises. The chilly, dark long periods of winter are an ideal time to get comfortable inside, with candles, toss covers, hot cocoa, wooly sweaters, and a good book or a TV show to gorge on. Loads of hygge nourishments, similar to flapjacks, porridge, and hot stew, are additionally perfect for winter.

In any case, that doesn't mean there's no space for hygge in the summer. Warm-climate hygge focuses more on outside exercises, for example, picnics, barbecues, blazes, or movie nights. Summertime hygge is about friendship and interfacing with nature, exploiting the warm climate while you can.

You can also characterize a hygge life by what it does not include. For example, going out to an in vogue move club, with flashing lights and pulsing electronic music, is about the most un-hygge action ever. Numerous other normal features of present-day life, for example, obsessively checking social media, going on a shopping binge at the shopping center, and eating inexpensive food, are additionally the exact opposite of hygge.

Chapter # 2

How the Hygge Life Can Save You Money

Unintentionally, hostile to hygge exercises like clubbing, eating out, and shopping also will, in general, share something different for all intents and purpose: they're costly. Hygge exercises, then again, will, in general, be modest or even free. That settles on the hygge way of life an ideal decision for enjoying a quality lifestyle on a tight budget.

Obviously, similar to some other pattern, hygge can be blamed for selling expensive items. Charlotte Higgins, writing for The Guardian, discusses seeing hygge "used to sell cashmere cardigans, wine, backdrop, veggie lover shepherd's pie, sewing designs, skincare extend, minuscule happy saddles for dachshunds, yoga withdraws and an occasion in a 'shepherd's cottage' in Kent." And obviously, there's no lack of books that you could burn through cash on to get familiar with hygge life.

But at its heart, hygge isn't about stuff. Rather, as story after story emphasizes, it's about a specific feeling or state of mind – something you can't get just by going through cash. Indeed, "futurist" Lucie Greene, addressing the New York Times, ventures to such an extreme as to call the hygge pattern a response against the prior "well-being movement," which appeared to focus on "$100 Lululemon tights and $10 bottles of cold-pressed juices."

The hygge way of life, paradoxically, is inside anybody's grasp. Like the voluntary simplicity movement, it centers around easing back down, grasping nature, and making more time for friends – everything you can manage without going through any cash whatsoever.

Hygge Happy

Presently you have a better understanding of what hygge is, yet what's the serious deal about carrying on with a hygge life? Without a doubt, we as a whole prefer to feel comfortable. However, is there additional to it? An answer may lie with the Danes. They have been embracing the hygge way of life for a very long time, to the point that it has become some portion of their national character. And, it appears to add to their general satisfaction factor. As indicated by the United

Nations World Happiness Report, Denmark is viewed as the happiest country in the world. This is somewhat amazing when you consider it. High expenses and long, cool winters with brief times of light aren't synonymous with happiness, as I would see it. But, the Danish people live contentedly practicing their hygge reasoning.

More than Candles, Homemade Cinnamon Rolls, and Cozy Decor

Indeed, these things can add to "hygge-ness," however, hygge life will change among us as people. For instance, I may love cookies simply out of the stove with gooey chocolate pieces while you may lean toward tasting spring cherry green tea from an ornamental porcelain teacup or a mug your child gave you (however it's alright to need a warm treat to go with it!).

Alongside a persistent enjoyment in comfortable things, hygge is likewise about convivial togetherness. A casual dinner with dear friends without heaps of complaint and a lot of well disposed of, agreeable cooperation is hygge. A personal favorite hygge fellowship minute for me is evening tea with my better half—our adaptation of a relaxed high tea. We sit in upholstered chairs with a perspective on the garden and drink fragrant tea saturated with hand-sewed silk tea sacks while buried in the discussion that wanders and spills out of point to the theme. Our lunchtimes together cultivate a deeper association between us.

Streamline and customize your space. It's hard to relax in overwhelming spaces. Clean up, evacuate additional things that don't satisfy you, and then surround yourself with objects that recount to a story—may be a framed image of you and a friend or family member or your pet, or a significant thing got during your movements.

Celebrating the High Hygge Season

Normally, the Christmas season is about hygge. Simply the idea of hot juice with a cinnamon stick and occasion music playing out of sight brings a cozy feeling. Sharing special moments and customs to loved ones and adding handcrafted gifts to your blessing trade— additionally hygge. Making a gift is fulfilling (and hygge) for both for you and the beneficiary, and it shouldn't be ultra-time-consuming. Make a terrarium or paint a wooden aviary you got up pastime store. Spot some hued glass beads in the base of Mason container, put a tea flame fair and level beads, tie a ribbon around the opening of the jar, and presto, you have a light holder that is incredible for a deck or a kitchen table.

Comfort food and evoking taste memories of glad

occasions in the past are hygge, as well. If it's very little whine, make your grandma's fudge, your dad's unique egg nog, or Auntie Sarah's freestyle plum tart.

Getting Hygge with the Neighbors

Neighborliness can be hygge. For example, my neighbor and I anticipate sharing what has become an annual tradition. It started when he hung a finch feeder that is obvious from our front doors. I contribute thistle seeds, as does he, to keep the "finch activity" going all through the season. My initial gift was planting moon roses, which reseed every year in a similar area as the bird feeder. We cheer when the seedlings grow, water the plants and watch them develop, at that point celebrate when their goliath white blooms spread out as nightfall moves close. (You may discover us out there doing a goofy impromptu moon move some night!) All this makes us feel great inside and supports a neighborly soul. Certainly hygge.

Practice appreciation. Cheer on a wonderful day by going on a bicycle ride or going for a walk. Welcome the bounty of goodness that originates from our neighborhood farms. Follow through a farmers market and get some crisp produce for you and your family to appreciate.

Simply thinking these things makes me "hygge happy." How about you?

APPROACHES TO LIVE HYGGE

In case you're keen on bringing somewhat more hygge into your life, there are bunches of approaches to do it at almost no expense. Here are a couple of thoughts:

1. Light Some Candles

Ask any Danish individual, and they'll reveal to you that the simplest method to make a hyggelig environment is with candles. Danes experience more candles than some other country on earth – an amazing 13 pounds of light wax per person every year. They even utilize the expression "lyselukker," which signifies "somebody who puts out the candles," to refer to a spoilsport.

Luckily, it's anything but difficult to find candles at deal costs. Stores like IKEA, Target, Bed Bath and beyond, and Amazon deliver enormous sacks of at any rate 100 tea lights for under $15. Try to utilize them securely: Don't put them on or approach anything flammable, keep them far from pets and little kids, and never leave a consuming flame unattended.

2. Light a Fire

If a tiny candle flame is comfortable, a fire is significantly cozier. It feels significantly more quick to watch a real fire than to have light and warmth delivered to you through electric bulbs and focal warming. In the late spring, you can gather around an open-air fire in an outside fire pit – lasting or convenient. In any event, cooking dinner over a grill barbecue allows you to watch the flames and possibly toast a couple of marshmallows.

In the winter, in case you're not lucky enough to have an indoor chimney, do the following best thing and stream a video of a crackling fire on your TV. You can't feel the warmth, yet you can even now watch the flames flicker and hear the logs pop. There are free chimney videos accessible on YouTube that run for three to 10 hours.

3. Put on Comfy Clothes

It's impossible to feel extremely comfortable while wearing a matching suit. To get hygge, you have to change into something simple and agreeable. Heavy sweaters and sewed socks are exemplary decisions for wintertime since they keep you warm, which is fundamental to the hygge state of mind. A couple of

Hyggebukser (sweats or different jeans you'd never wear openly) complete the outfit.

4. Take a Walk

Danes love to take long walks in a wide range of climate – whatever may happen, winter or summer. Walking is particularly hyggelig when you do it with a friend or a group of friends. It's an opportunity to talk and appreciate each other's conversation without spending a penny. But, in any event, going for a walk all alone, or with your dog, is an approach to draw nearer to nature and enjoy a break from a busy schedule.

5. Ride a Bike

Bikes are famous in Denmark. Denmark.dk, the country's official site, says the capital city of Copenhagen is known for its cycling society and is perceived as the main authority Bike City on the planet. Bicycles are hygge because they move at a slower pace than vehicles, allowing you to enjoy the view. If you effectively possess a bicycle, think about cycling to work. Various studies show that people who bicycle to work are both more beneficial and happier than individuals who drive. In case you don't have one, check whether you can get one used. Sites like Craigslist and eBay regularly have fundamental models in great condition for $100 or less. Another choice is to join a bicycle sharing system if your city has one.

6. Offer a Meal

Home cooking is considerably more hyggelig than eating out, and it's doubly so if you share the meal with a couple of old buddies. To make your dinner party as hygge as could be allowed, center around comfort food as opposed to haute cuisine. Fresh and common fixings are acceptable, yet an extravagant introduction is pointless. Well, known dishes for Danes incorporate pancakes, meatballs, and rice cakes, yet you can serve whatever feels generally comforting to you – regardless of whether that is your mom's chicken soup or your preferred apple crumble. If cooking for a group is more work than you can deal with, hold a potluck. That way, every one of your friends can bring their preferred cozy dishes and offer them, which knocks up the hygge remainder significantly more.

7. Drink Something Hot

The quintessential hygge drink in Denmark is glögg or spiced thought about wine. In any case, basically any hot drink – coffee, tea, hot chocolate – can add to a hyggelig environment. On a cool, wet day, there's nothing cozier than sitting inside with a steaming mug in your grasp, and it's a pleasure that costs just pennies.

8. Read a Book

Reading is a hygge action since it's a method to slow down and detach yourself from the occupied, quick-paced current world. You can up the hygge factor by curling up on a lounge chair with your book and a blanket, or in a hotter climate, sitting outside to read under a tree.

9. Watch TV with Friends

Sitting in front of the TV can likewise be a hygge movement, especially if you do it with companions. Scary shows are an especially hygge decision, insofar as they're fictional; it feels additional comfortable to watch something alarming when you know you're protected and cozy in your home. Danes particularly love police procedurals about deranged killers.

The greatest hit show of this sort was "Forbrydelsen," which gave viewers a good scare as well as brought forth a whole site, SarahLundSweater.com, gave to the substantial, designed fleece sweater worn by the female analyst. (An American adjustment of this arrangement, called "The Killing," is available on Netflix.) Stick to fictional alarms, in any case, watching something frightening; for example, and the news makes the wrong mood completely.

10. Play Board Games

Hosting a tabletop game night is also a very hygge approach to go through the night. Tabletop games offer an approach to play around with friends at home at little cost and with no fancy technology. This ticks off three of the hygge boxes: companionship, relaxation, and simplicity.

11. Sing Songs

Having a sing-along in your home may seem like something straight out of the 1960s; however, in Denmark, it's as yet a common action. "The Book of Hygge," noticed that numerous Danish family units have copies of a society songbook, and they sing from it to "avow the thoughts of simplicity, cheerfulness, reciprocity, community and belonging." If you'd prefer to check out this, a great American equivalent this book is "Ascend singing," which contains lyrics and harmonies for a wide range of singable songs, from customary people to the Beatles to Tin Pan Alley.

12. Snuggle

What action might be cozier than snuggling? It consolidates about all the components of hygge – comfort, relaxation, simplicity, and spending time with individuals you're near – in one. Cuddle under a cover with your friend, your children, your closest friend, your pet – or every one of them simultaneously. It's warm and happy, and it costs nothing by any stretch of the imagination.

HYGGE MANIFESTO

Except if you have been living in a cave, you more likely than not knew about the Danish idea of Hygge. It is tied in with getting a charge out of the ordinary, network, comfort, and feeling better. It is the Danish lifestyle, an action word, a thing, and an excellent method to acknowledge life.

My partner has been a specialist of Hygge for a long time. She found it when contemplating why Denmark is constantly appraised as the happiest country. We met several years back, and she convinced me to check out it as the evenings got darker, and the climate began to make me take a look at cheap flights to exotic countries. I have never been in winter. I realize a few people love getting comfortable and wearing wool; it was simply never my thing. I like daylight, being warm, and being barefoot. I need to state, however, that Hygge has truly helped me to appreciate winter specifically yet additionally more by and large, life. It is eventually about being glad, and I find that practicing Hygge has made me happier.

As should be obvious, over the manifesto calls for us to be available at the time truly and completely draw in with life. By achieving physical comfort, interfacing with others (not on a screen), being thankful, and making a delightful environment, we can achieve Hyggelig emotions. These are feelings of security and happiness that emerge from your sensory experiences.

This is the reason Hygge focuses on climate, making a soothing space in which to relax is significant. It additionally necessitates that we set aside an effort to discover and appreciate pleasurable things — don't surge some tea, take as much time as is needed and enjoy the taste and the warmth of the cup in your embrace. You don't have to go through cash to do Hygge, and it isn't just about Scandi interiors. It is about your mentality to life and how much attention you pay to get a charge out of everything.

I surmise this all sounds comfortable, and if you are working 60 hours every week and have a bustling family unit or a lot of stress, this may all sound a little fantastic. I can't help disagreeing, however. Sure it is simpler to enjoy life when you have a lot of time; however, even in my most focused on times I realize, I could have found more time to appreciate something little, and that would have had any effect. We, as a whole, need to deal with ourselves. Here and there, that can be a couple of little things which truly mean feeling better and being more able to manage life's pressures. Next time you are worn out and reach to turn the television on, why not try simply tuning in to some music or getting your friends and family together for a game of cards. I know when we are destroyed by energy, these things can appear to be unthinkable; however, they are impossible, despite all the trouble. Consider how much time you spend staring at a screen and see if you can discover 30 minutes to do something else this week.

Approaches to Bring Hygge into Your Home

Does your home cause you to feel warm and comfortable? When you return home around evening time, do you get a feeling of peace and tranquility from your environment? Truly, you should.

Our homes are an individual expansion of ourselves, so

when you stroll through the front door, you should feel relaxed and quiet. In case you're not, it's the ideal opportunity for the family to do what the Danes do and embrace Hygge.

Hygge (articulated: Hoo-Gah) is the Danish idea of making a comfortable air in your home. As indicated by Marty Basher, Home Organization Expert for Modular Closets, Hygge is additionally the confirmation of a feeling or moment.

Considering United Nations World Happiness Report records Denmark as one of the happiest countries on the planet, and we figure those content Danish might be on to something with their journey for Hygge!

In any case, bringing the Hygge idea into your home doesn't mean a total renovation. There are basic approaches to make your home more comfortable.

Here are a few different ways you can fuse Hygge into your environment:

1. Replace Harsh Lights

Utilize delicate lights or darker lampshades to dispose of brilliant lighting, or think about lighting candles around your home. (In case you're stressed over open flares, try LED candles.) Candles and delicate lighting produce a calming mood, says Hygge master Bee Heinemann. "The thought is to make a space that looks and feels softer, quieter, and more relaxing."

2. Cook at Home

Hygge cooking is about comfort food, warm, healthy dishes that cause you to feel all comfortable inside. And, cooking them as a family makes it Hygge-is (would we be able to state that?).

Says Heinemann, doing this, sets aside cash, is more advantageous, and bonds the family when they're sitting around the kitchen table. "Empower family support in dinner arranging, nourishment prep, and cooking. At whatever point a kid has contributed to meal preparation, they are more disposed to need to eat what they've cooked."

3. Promote Relaxation in the Home

Stress should drift away the moment you enter your home. (Alright, more difficult than one might expect, yet at least try.)

Bad day at outside? Proceed forward, and set aside a few minutes for yourself and your family, says Heinemann. "Express great morning and a great night to your friends and family, make sure to get some information about their day or to state 'good luck' on that test. Give embraces when you leave and return home."

Additionally, detach from hardware, online networking, and TV. Think about covering your TV with a pretty texture when not being used; its energy can be an interruption.

Ask yourself: Do you truly need to check your cell phone constantly?

4. Conquer Your Clutter

"Completely embracing Hygge means conquering mess," says Marty Basher. "Mess is an outward expression of an absence of thinking about something in your life. It might be a side-effect of a missing self-care routine or misalignment of needs inside the time you have. Embrace Hygge by assessing the root cause(s) of the clutter in your home and care for them. As you care for those, the clutter clears, and the visual proof of the Hygge feeling can be seen."

Think twice about bringing 'random' things into a little home. Do you truly require another mermaid/mustache/bacon thing? Each item that enters a little home, says Basher, must have direction and be thought about, or it reduces the feeling of cozy invitation.

"Keep up Hygge in a little home by picking things that are both functional and sentimental, remembering the inclination you will have when you bring it home." Will the thing add to the sentiment of care and solace in your home, or become clutter?

5. Organize With Bins and Baskets

Utilize natural crates or bins in warm color to compose after you clean up.

"Expel everything without a down to earth reason or the stuff that doesn't add to the general look of your home," echoes Lily Cameron, Cleaning, and Hygge Expert at Fantastic Services. "Put resources into helpful coordinators, and your place will look more spacious and organized. Expelling the cluttered mess around will assist you with keeping your psyche clear and assist you with achieving inner peace...?"

Concerning dens, Cameron says store toys in various named boxes and containers. "You won't just sort out the play area yet make the child's activity a lot simpler with regards to taking the toys back to their right spot."

6. Surround Yourself with Happiness

It's alright to bring a few things into your home, however, ensure they're sentimental things that bring out happy memories, says Heinemann, resounding Basher's thoughts.

"Think framed photographs or fine art, a jar with shells, a delightful stone gathered from the sea, a bowl of your distant grandma's, or something you got on your travels abroad."

7. Bring Nature Indoors

"Plants make the air fresh, and their green color is a solution for our eyes and nerves," says Cameron. "Improve your place by putting more plants inside the home. This will also make the room brighter and cozier and let you inhale far more new and clean air."

8. Think about Music and Aromas

Hygge isn't constantly about the inside, stresses Cameron. "Hygge must be felt with our different faculties, as well." Along with the visual pleasure, including some ambient music and smells to your home will also improve the home air—as long as the aroma or music is soothing and not overbearing.

9. Use Soothing Colors and Textures

In case you need to go hard and fast, Hygge, consider repainting your space. Check out your home and truly take in its color plan, room by room. Do the colors feel welcoming? As indicated by Vänt Wall Panels, Interior Design Expert Bee Heinemann, a home with soothing shades and soft textures sets the general mindset.

"Think peaceful blues, greens, grays, whites, and beiges," she says, and settle on delicate furniture with adjusted edges and hardwood floors with soft area rugs.

Chapter # 3

How to Hygge:

The possibility of Hygge is to be available at the time you're in, and aware of how to make THIS minute one that you can love. While researching the, what/why/when/how of this thought, there were a couple of things that truly stood out to me. These were:

Being Present:

Being discontent is simple, and it falls into place without any issues. Without avoiding a beat, I could list 5-10 things I wish were different at present. How about we do something somewhat harder, and pause for a minute to clear the mind and truly center on the present time and place. Take a full breath and be at the time, list 5-10 things you're appreciative for now. Work on being at the time and loving the moment.

I could without much of a stretch go through my morning daydreaming about spring and all the things I'm arranging and loving about THAT season. Yet, this habit possibly breeds unhappy emotions when I "come to" and recall that it's still January. To be my happiest self, I'm working on being available and loving this moment.

Being Intentional:

Everything around you and everything that you do, add to your day and makes it either great, bad, or in the middle. Being purposeful about making your day can affect a good or bad day. The little things count!

Something as basic as setting aside the effort to light a scented flame or planning something for changing the environment around yourself for the better can affect between a "blah day" and a good day.

Being intentional about the environment in your home, the exercises you do, the food you eat, and the music you tune in to-would all be able to mean a happier, cozier time.

How I've been deliberate about my day:

I began progressing in the direction of having a good day since the minute I woke up. It is anything but an idiot-proof arrangement; however, a culture of making steps that you realize will cause you to feel great. I began my day by drinking a glass of water-a demonstration that causes me to feel great truly, yet additionally helps wake me up and feel alert. Which is significant because I am NOT a morning person! This was my method for giving the morning. It's the best chance.

My following stage was to put on some happy music and start my oil diffuser with a mix of "Peace" and Lavender basic oils. As I prepared for my day, I went over my daily psychological agenda and included little ways I could make the day more enjoyable. It shouldn't be hard; for me, it's as basic as adding scents and sounds to the environment in my home to feel cozier.

Another method for organizing joy is to be more intentional about self-care. For me, this means booking time to do yoga and take a walk. Yoga is relaxing, and taking a walk gives personal time to appreciate daylight and outside air. The two exercises give a touch of energy to my progression and light up the day. Consider what lights up your day and cause you to feel incredible; at that point, organize those things.

Saying Yes/Indulge Yourself:

Something I continued going over while finding out about Hygge was simply reveling. It's tied in with focusing on what may present to you a measure of comfort or joy and saying yes to that. From nourishment, drinks, comfortable sweaters, or anything sensibly speaking, you can consider making the season lovely. Do those things, eat those foods, and say yes to yourself.

Get Outside:

Spending time outdoors is beneficial for us, truly and emotionally! I am bad at this in the winter, and I loathe the virus! My objective this winter is to be better about getting outside. Although it's cold, get out there and get some natural air. Set aside some effort to get what little daylight peeks out this season, and fill your lungs with some great natural air. This consistently fills in as a great pick-me-up. Dress properly for the climate and go on a walk.

Be/Do/Create Cozy

In all that you do this season, make comfortable. There are such huge numbers of approaches to do this! Pause for a minute to think about the things that cause you to feel warm and fuzzy inside. This rundown may incorporate things like: spending time with friends/family, playing prepackaged games, nestling up under a cover with tea and a good book, going sledding with your kids, preparing and eating uncommon treats, taking a day to give your home a comfortable/warm environment, the list goes on. Organize this, be intentional about being comfortable.

Hygge isn't Hard

As we've learned through this post, hygge isn't a difficult practice to employ. For all the potential advantages of implementing these methods, it requires remarkably little effort. As occupied spouses and moms, the estimation of such simple yet happiness-inducing systems can be endless.

This year, I challenge myself as well as every one of you to do at any rate one hygge roused action for each day. To assist with this test, I've made the greatest and best hygge list ever, which you can discover in the resource library!

THE MOST EFFECTIVE METHOD TO HYGGE WITH A BABY

Hygge with a q as much as possible from this season. One of my top personal choices approaches to beat the winter blues is by implementing Hygge into my day by day life. This year I find a good pace, my child!

Get Cozy!

Hygge is an extraordinary method to remain feeling

cozy and glad throughout the winter months and all year! Anyway, similarly, as with all things, your way of life changes when you have an infant in the home. One thing that changes is getting more intentional with your time. A portion of your old most loved approaches to loosen up perhaps a little unrealistic as a mother (who has the opportunity to twist up with a good book, or wash up? Not me!). As mothers, we're occupied, and a few days, the main time we may spend sitting down is while taking care of the child.

A year ago, I spent my winter implementing Hygge while pregnant and impatiently anticipating the appearance of my first little girl. This year, I'm figuring out how to Hygge with a baby! Go along with me on my journey and read on for extraordinary tips on the most proficient method to comfortable up with your child close behind.

Take advantage of every moment

Regardless of whether you're simply sitting down for some time to take care of your child, set aside 5 minutes in front of the effort to plan.

- Get a glass of water or potentially tea, coffee, or hot cocoa

- Light a scented candle or get some great scents

moving (oil diffuser or Scentsy hotter?)

- Put on some music

- Pick up your preferred book or diversion while nursing

Try not to leave this time alone a chore, cuddle your child while you feed her, and taste your favorite drink. This is your opportunity to "look at" for a moment and forget your different tasks. Taking care of the child is a need, and you have the chance to make a comfortable environment while you do as such!

Make Cozy

Spend a little time reflecting the things that fulfill you, what sparks joy? What things cause you to feel warm and comfortable inside?

- Be deliberate about "reveling" in what fulfills you. Regardless of whether it's loading up on your preferred tea and hot cocoa, dressing child in cute outfits only for ordinary, or decorating for Christmas on Nov. 1!

- Lighting is everything! It's said that Denmark (where Hygge begins!) consumes a greater number of candles than some other nation. I know I would say having a light lit in the room sparks comfortable and warm feelings!

In case you have little youngsters, make certain to put any candles in a safe spot, or settle on a more secure option, for example, electric candles as well as scents hotter for that same subtle lighting effect.

Put thought into your spaces

Consider where you invest the vast majority of your energy; is it in the parlor? Kitchen? Playroom? Or, on the other hand, the schoolroom if you self-teach? Organize making this space agreeable for you. This can mean anything from making an agreeable spot to sit and take care of a child, to an assigned day by day brief clean up right now keep it clean and uncluttered.

Hygge at night is my top choice, and I know without a doubt, my child nods off simpler when the lights are turned down, flame lit, and a soft piano lullaby playlist on. I'm loose, and along these lines, she relaxes and falls asleep!

Manage Expectations

This might be your first winter/Christmas season with a baby, and it will be for me! So I'm trying to get ready by being simple with myself about what's sensible.

Here's how I'm doing that:

- Identify your baby's needs. My child needs to be sleeping by 7, and that is something I need to remember when taking her places. Have some good times and go to occasion family social affairs, however, remember those requirements. A child will at present be drained at 7, although we're at grandmas! Arrange how to deal with those requirements.

- Be OK with saying "no" to welcomes. Family Christmas? No doubt I plan on going to that, however the yearly Christmas eve party?

Presumably not going to make it, because family cuddles and getting the child to bed on time is more important to me! I realize that early, so I'm dealing with my desires.

Enjoy your home time!

Nothing is more Hygge than getting a charge out of comfortable occasions with your friends and family at home. Make hot chocolate, cuddle up by the fire, and appreciate delighting in the delight of the family this winter. My heart is never happier than when I'm cuddled up viewing a decent film with my children and Husband.

Hygge and Baby

The special seasons can be unpleasant, and a long winter with a baby may appear to be daunting to a few. In any case, lets Hygge it out! This is my girl's first winter, and by implementing Hygge with her and developing an atmosphere of love, warmth, and friendliness, I plan to instill traditions of comfortable winters from now through adulthood.

By being intentional today, we are making recollections that our kids will think back on affectionately.

Feeling Hygge

You've likely heard the term before, regardless of whether the definition was unclear. That is because hygge—a Danish word without an immediate English translation—is somewhat difficult to portray. In any case, we're going to try. Hygge (articulated "hoo-ga") intends to recognize a feeling or minute that is comfortable, charming, or special. A closer translation is something much the same as "too comfortable around together." The word isn't new; however, more as of late specialists have made a translated of hygge into a method for child-rearing, a Danish way of life that fits bringing up cheerful, skilled children.

So how might you grasp hygge at home? The thought

is to spend a great deal of calm quality time together, free of distractions. There is additionally a positive emphasis on getting comfortable and sustaining familial bonds through physical and emotional connections.

For what reason do we give it a second thought? The Danish have made a reputation for being the happiest people on Earth, so if satisfaction is the objective, we may have some things to learn.

Start Small

Similarly, as with anything, embracing another way of life, or right now perspective doesn't occur at the same time. For some, choosing a couple of Danish child-rearing thoughts and standards will be sufficient. Others may choose to all the more completely incorporate this idea into their life after some time.

Start by picking a couple of thoughts or suggestions that support a feeling of hygge. At that point, put those by and by. As the first round of thoughts starts to feel like the new ordinary, include a couple more or increase the time you spend moving in the direction of hygge, continually modifying it to your family's individual needs and preferences.

Indeed, even as you progress, hygge is never something

to be done day in and day out. Hygge is finding peace in minutes, not throughout the day regular. Indeed, even the Danes don't feel hygge that much. Also, to that point, after some time, hygge ought to be, to a lesser extent, conscious practice and even more thought and schedule. It's accepted that individuals in Denmark don't place a great deal of thought into finding hygge; rather, it is a feeling that is ingrained in them through routine exercises that promote hygge.

Getting a handle on the Intangible

Hygge is best described as a believing, a psychological state, and an inner peace. This makes turning into a hygge family a little gray. There isn't just one activity that embraces hygge; rather, there are a few alternatives that make a feeling of hygge in your family unit.

From numerous points of view, hygge is tied in with associating with your kids. It includes giving your full attention (not generally, yet in these quiet, still minutes), doing something comfortable together, and embracing not being occupied. At its center, hygge advances a feeling of calmness that children and adults both respond to.

Hygge doesn't mean you need to sit idle. Rather, search for exercises that are unstructured and should be possible as a family. Connect while doing, however, don't over arrangement since then you end up forgoing the "save time" some portion of the idea that advances that inner quiet we wish we had as parents—and our youngsters as non-domesticated animals—both had.

Set aside a few minutes

Cut out little pieces of the day or week to take part in exercises that encourage hygge. For instance, pick one night of the week to be a family night where everybody returns home at a respectable hour and spends time alone together.

During tonight put the PDAs away, don't answer work calls or messages, and pick an action that empowers holding, may it paint, viewing a film, or playing tabletop games. There are only a couple (free) rules. Everything must be done together, the action ought to be sensibly quiet, and during the action, you should find time to associate either physically, emotionally, or mentally.

Get Started

- Attempt a portion of these errands.

- Sip hot cocoa before a fire

- Wear nightwear in the day or early night

- Get agreeable and close with covers and sweaters

- Turn off the screens and discuss over tea

- Eat supper on the lounge chair and cuddle while viewing a film

- Play tabletop games by candlelight

- Bake or cook together

Why Kids Like It

Hygge energizes individuals—like excessively busy Americans—to set aside some effort to back off. In these minutes, the emphasis is on building intimacy with others. Kids like it when parents slow down and focus on family; it can assist kids with feeling heard and loved. This, thus, makes an inner peace and certainty that will assist kids with thriving throughout everyday life. It additionally sets them up to find that equivalent peace and stillness amid find as they grow, and ideally share similar beliefs and standards with future families. That is the reason it works for the Danes; they don't know about hygge because it is a lifestyle to them. Hygge will, in general, conflict with a portion of the standards American families are utilized to. For instance, hygge requests families to be less occupied and to give in to quiet, maybe unstructured, time as a family. While in America, we promote enrichment exercises and extracurricular, hygge is doing without these needs (here and there) for something more serene.

The exercises that lead to hygge explicitly take into account finding quiet and building associations with others. Hygge doesn't include yelling or drama, and it is the capacity to shed that pressure and negativity at the door and rather interface. Yet, hygge isn't just for families; it works for friends and adults, too.

Hygge Techniques Everyone Should Try For a Cozy Home

You likely observe the buzzy term "hygge" on your preferred way of life writes or hear it on an HGTV design show, and wonder what the hell hygge is about. The Danish way of life pattern brings out feelings of warmth and is about comfort; however, if you are carrying on with a fast-paced modernized life (particularly with kids!), it might feel hard to discover approaches to fuse hygge into your everyday life. These eight hygge methods everybody should read a comfortable home are anything but difficult to do, and can help get you started to find the true soul of hygge living.

I'd you are not effectively acquainted with the hygge pattern of carrying on with a simplified, snuggly life, prepare to get ready for the idea. Helen Russell, a British columnist and top of the line creator of The Year of Living Danishly — Uncovering The Secrets of the World's Happiest Country, experienced directly what hygge is and how it is lived in the real culture where it started. "The word defies literal translation yet the best clarification I've found in over six years of living danishly is 'the finished absence of anything irritating or emotionally overpowering: taking delight from the presence of delicate, relieving things.'"

Ahhh. Don't you feel cozier simply hearing that definition? Read on for approaches to incorporate hygge in your home and help make a comfortable space where you can enjoy happy, merry minutes between your baby's inevitable meltdowns.

1. Comfortable Activities

Most importantly, understanding that hygge isn't just about how your house is decorated can improve things greatly in embracing the way of life. Pia Edberg, creator of The Cozy Life: Rediscover the Joy of the Simple

Things through the Danish Concept of Hygge, discloses to Romper that hygge is "considerably more than physical or aesthetic comfort." Regardless of how you may improve your home, Edberg clarifies that comfortable exercises additionally assume a role in making a hygge situation. "It's additionally about mental and emotional wellbeing and surrounding yourself with individuals and things that you love, and that causes you to feel protected, warm, and comfortable. It's also about doing comfortable exercises, for example, reading a decent book with some tea, having a good discussion with a friend or group of friends, or a cuddle with a hairy pet. With hygge, we create comfort, intimacy, and connection."

2. Warm Lighting

Russell takes note of that candlelight is one of the more significant parts of hygge living and clarifies how it is normally done in Danish culture. "Candlelight is a key part (Danes consume the most significant number of candles per head in Europe.) And they're all over: from the windowsill of my children's childcare to shops, banks," Russell says. "Hygge is so significant to living danishly that I once observed a camper van driving along with the engine with lit candles in the windows. This is likely illegal, yet Vikings don't will, in general, be too hung up on well-being and security."

Although the vast majority of us keep an eye on the flip on a light switch when we have to illuminate our homes, experts state that making a hygge environment in your house is as simple as lighting a few candles or changing your bulbs. "Hygge lighting is comfortable, warm, reduce, yellow in tone," Edberg tells Romper. "So if you can get dimmers on your lights, utilize yellow conditioned lights, light candles, hang pixie lights — these will make your space super comfortable when lit up when it's dark outside."

3. Get the Outdoors

Russell says that the Danes normally utilize numerous characteristic components inside their homes to make a hygge situation. She says that "wood, cowhide, [and] sheepskin floor coverings" are basic components that the Danish utilize that can also be. Incorporated to make your own home feel more hygge.

Edberg additionally prescribes gathering characteristic components that carry the outside into your home to make it cozier. "We normally feel quiet when we are surrounded ordinarily, so get lots of plants or blossoms from outside to enable you to relax," Edberg says. "You can assemble a bundle of wild roses to place in your home, or some interesting bits of driftwood, or rocks/precious stones."

4. Comfortable Textiles

Russell clarifies that comfort is key with regards to hygge-inspired materials, particularly during the virus winter months, when the hygge association is at its peak. "Couches will, in general, have a comfortable blanket thrown over the rear of them during this season and come with a wealth of pads — Danes pay attention to their comfort very," Russell tells Romper.

You also don't need to put resources into anything costly to make the materials in your home hygge. "Discover materials that make you need to twist up in them," Edberg says. "You can take whatever blankets/pillows you effectively possess and put them out in plain view around the house, on the couches/seats, kitchen, office, and so forth."

5. Calming Colors

To make your home more hygge, switching up your color plan might be an interesting point if your home features all the more brightly colored items or wall paint. In Danish culture, Russell clarifies that planned colors are delicate and propelled naturally. "Hues are serene and stylishly planned," Russell tells Romper. "So there's been a major pattern in grays and pale salmon pinks, yet this year we're seeing increasingly olive greens and quieted, organically inspired colors."

With hygge, you can dim our light in coloring inside your home, as long as the coloring plan is relieving to you. "I think whether one picks lighter colors (pastel hues) or darker colors (deep reds/purple/green/blues) relies upon individual taste, yet I would avoid anything too bright, energetic, or jarring like neon colors," Edberg says. "Fundamentally, if you can cause your space to feel like a comfortable spa or a comfortable lodge escape (whatever your taste is), it will feel hygge to you."

6. Communicate

Edberg recommends that mirroring your style by showing things of individual significance in your home can be a type of hygge. "You need your space to feel like you. It could be photographs of you and your friends/family, or a puppet you got on your movements, or your works of art hung up on the wall in case you're an artist. Show these, don't tuck them," Edberg tells Romper.

7. Partake In Self-Care

Although it may not seem like something that will make your physical home cozier, taking part in hygge ideas that inspire self-care can help put you in a hygge mentality, which will thus permit you to all the more completely connect with when making your home a more hygge space.

"Spend some hygge time with yourself, reduce the lights, put on certain candles and delicate, relaxing music (quieting music is hygge!), and give yourself some self-esteem, similar to a hot shower, reflecting, reading a good book with some tea, or nestling with a pet," Edberg says. "At last hygge is about a feeling, instead of a visual stylish. You can hygge anyplace as it's everything about the mentality and the love you put into a minute. It's about not deciding on anybody or anything, and allowing individuals to have a sense of security as who they seem to be, while also feeling relaxed and comfortable."

8. Welcome Others into Your Home

Experts explain that to make your home a hygge situation, you should fill it with friends and friends and family to take part in hygge exercises, particularly in the colder months. "Hygge is tied up with the climate, which has a holding impact," Russell says. "It's so cold and dull October to March that everybody meets up. In hotter atmospheres, you can even now go out and spend time in restaurants and cafes, however living danishly means you arrange at home and get hygge."

When you have made your home a hygge haven, welcoming others over to partake in the space together is vital. "I think one about the greatest things we can do, particularly with the digital age diverting us, is deliberately making association and time with our loved ones or companions/family," Edberg says. "Do something personal and not very overstimulation — like appreciating hot cocoa and having a good catch-up conversation. Hygge is antiquated, loose, and not particular."

Chapter # 4

Instructions to Get Through a Miserable Winter

For a few, the winter is a magical season. For others like me, it's a gloomy, cold, darkness you need to hold up out. Yet, there's a superior method to get past winter. An outlook that includes embracing the one of a kind parts of the winter months. Enter the Danish idea of "hygge."

Hygge, which is an expression of Norwegian beginning, is articulated "hoo-gah" and freely means "comfort." But while comfort is a significant bit of the puzzle, hygge is extremely a greater amount of an attitude or mindset. As Natalie Van Deusen, teacher of Scandinavian Studies at the University of Alberta puts it:

"The best translation is comfort, yet not the physical comfort that you get when you put on a sweater or cuddle up with a cover. It's, even more, a state mental parity and mental health."

It's a feeling a large number of us feel when we return home for holidays. In any case, it doesn't have left when you head back to the real world. Furthermore, trust me, the Danish hear what they're saying. They have the absolute longest, harshest winters, yet they're perhaps the happiest countries in the world. Here are a few hints on how you can achieve hygge this winter and ideally appreciate it more than expected.

Double Down On Coziness

It may not be the genuine meaning of hygge, yet getting truly comfortable can, in any case, help. Fundamentally, I become a specialist at digging in at home and getting as agreeable as could be expected under the circumstances. Reading a book by the fire with a hot drink is hygge. So is eating natively constructed prepared merchandise while sitting in front of the TV under a pile of covers. You can never have enough blankets, pillows, warm socks, hot drinks, or cuddling with your pet or significant other.

To achieve a definitive comfortable environment, Susanne Nilsson, a teacher on the Danish language at Morley College, recommends you mind the space around you. It's ideal to avoid huge, void rooms, just as spaces that look cold. Dump the fluorescent lights and utilize different kinds of lighting to further your potential benefit to cause huge rooms to feel smaller and hotter. Meik Wiking, the writer of The Little Book of Hygge, suggests you light huge amounts of candles, use lights with warm, soft-lit bulbs, and get a fire moving in the fireplace if you have one. If not, even a TV with a phony fireplace video can help. It's everything about changing your home to coordinate the style of the period, so it feels like an impenetrable post of happiness and warmth.

Consider wintering your opportunity to rest and your warm home as your bear cavern. Blame the winter to do those things you've been putting off. Nestle up on the sofa lastly finish that book, remain under your spreads and get past that TV show everybody has been discussing, or hop in the shower and listen in to your backlog of podcasts. Do those things you won't possess energy for once the climate clears up, and you need to go outside. I've been investing more energy in my comfortable bed, tasting great coffee, reading books, and playing Vita games I haven't completed at this point.

Assemble With Good Company as regularly as possible

The winter regularly reduces the measure of time you go through with others. Harsh cool, foul climate, and risky streets make social affairs and outings an issue. But, friendship and friendliness are a fundamental part of hygge, and the Danish think keeping up strong social associations is useful for the soul.

There are two approaches to hygge-style get-togethers. To begin with, you can sort out normal, relaxed meetups with friends or family at somebody's home with snacks, treats, and delicious drinks. Helen Russell, the creator of The Year of Living Danishly: Uncovering the Secrets of the World's Happiest Country, recommends these social occasions are tied in with simply reveling and making some good memories. So welcome your friends over, have some cake, coffee, juice, doughnuts, or whatever you like, and simply spending time talking in your comfortable front room and appreciating each other's conversation. Often should you do this as much as possible? Star tip: break out the occasional things to truly embrace what the winter brings to the table. Lagers, treats, and whatever else that is selective to this season.

If you don't have a comfortable home, you can have hygge-style social events in comfortable cafés, bars, cafes, or even book shops. Try not to let those comfortable lounge chairs at the neighborhood café go to waste. My friends and I like prepackaged game cafes, where you can keep warm, have coffee, and play huge amounts of games for cheap. Furthermore, in case you're all alone in another spot, the Lonely Planet Guide to Copenhagen recommends hygge members don't need to be people, you know. Post up at a cozy cafe or bar and try to make some new friends.

Appreciate Winter Wonderlands in the Right Gear

I hate being cold and wet, so I don't care about going out in the day off the freezing wind. Also, thus, I've never put resources into good winter clothing. Might it be able to be that I detest being exposed to the harsh elements of reality basically because I've kept myself from being appropriately arranged for it? If I bought some decent winter garments, and they kept me warm, perhaps I'd appreciate it... Because it's freezing out doesn't mean you needn't bother with a little action, regardless of whether it's only a walk. Get a good coat, pair of gloves, boots, caps, snow pants, whatever you have to step outside, and feel 100% great. Once more, not "sufficiently warm," 100% agreeable.

What's more, when you do head outside, consider doing exercises you can do throughout the winter. It could be skiing, snowboarding, ice skating, sledding, or having a snowball fight. Try to value the exercises, sights, and sounds you can understand during this season, and you'll only experience during this time of year, and you'll stop wishing it was summer already.

Slow Down and Find Joy In the Little Things

Wiking summarizes the essence of hygge as "the quest for everyday happiness." It's utilizing the winter a long time to focus on the basic joys throughout everyday life, take a stab at relaxation and comfort, and seek after harmony consistently. At the point when you take a look at winter through a viewpoint like that, it feels a lot hotter. Who knows? You may even begin to miss winter come springtime.

HYGGE CHRISTMAS!

Make a comfortable Hygge Christmas with our tips and lot s. Christmas is the ideal time to rehearse and appreciate Hygge!

Hygge (hoo-guh) is tied in with being content, comfortable, and getting a charge out of the simple and little things throughout everyday life. This Danish word and lifestyle are difficult to explain appropriately. It is best characterized by how you feel when you do something.

Hygge is tied in with being warm and comfortable. It is

tied in with being with loved ones or alone. It is tied in with having a comfortable home and room, doing comfortable exercises, and simply getting a charge out of the basic things. Hygge is a method for getting things done and how you feel doing those things.

Christmas is the ideal time for Hygge. Since Christmas (ought to be) tied in with being with individuals, you love and like, great food and drink, comfortable indoor exercises, and feeling warm and content.

Such a significant number of the things that we as a whole love about Christmas are also so beloved of Hygge. This incorporates candles, genuine flames, warm sweaters, and hot soothing drinks.

Hygge is tied in with being warm inside when it is cold outside. It is tied in with appreciating food and drink that warms and fills us. It is about social occasions of individuals and enjoying simple pleasures and traditions.

Truly there is no closure to the Hygge you can make during the Christmas season. Winter is the absolute best time for Hygge, as it fits the feel of warm and comfortable that we feel inside when the climate is cold, and it is dark outside.

Here are a few recommendations for making a Hygge

Christmas this year!

1. Candles and Lights

Candles and lights are so ideal for both Hygge and Christmas. They make a warm glow. Candles give off a glow and make your home smell dazzling. Lights put out a shine and liven up something dark.

Your Christmas tree is the ideal spot for lights. String lights all around your Christmas tree. There is nothing more excellent during the Christmas season than killing all your other house lights, and simply sitting taking a look at a lit Christmas tree.

Light candles on your mantelpiece, and your coffee table. Purchase candles that have the aromas of the period. These incorporate fragrances, for example, cinnamon, pine, cranberry, and berries.

Turn off your electric powered lights and appreciate the delicate shine of candles. They make an all the more smooth, comfortable light, rather than the brash electric lights.

2. Baking

Baking is the ideal thing for Hygge and Christmas. In addition to the fact that it is agreeable to prepare and spend time making something, it additionally makes your home smell pretty wonderful!

Preparing Christmas treats, for example, gingerbread treats, and more will put magnificent smells all-around you are home.

You can share your baking with your family and visitors. Any engaging is such a great amount of better with great food and drink.

Make baking a major piece of your Hygge Christmas.

3. Get the Outside

Nature is a major piece of Hygge. Nature is additionally so common all through the Christmas season. It is the one genuine season when we don't think twice about bringing a tree inside!

Having a Christmas tree is one of the most magnificent approaches to bring nature into your home. Taking a gander at nature and the outside makes calm thoughts and emotions in us.

If you feel awful about having a real Christmas tree – and truly there is nothing so uncommon as having that real tree up at Christmas time with its exceptional smell, consider purchasing a tree with a ball root so that you can replant it after Christmas.

Wreaths are additionally an awesome method for acquiring the outside. Spot a wreath on your front door, on your mantelpiece, and anyplace else in your home. You need some greenery. Wreaths are anything but difficult to make with only a couple of pine branches.

You can be as insignificant as you need to with including nature inside. Only a couple of pine branches in a vase on your table can instill a superb feeling of the outdoors and nature.

4. Make your Home Cozy and Comfortable

Hygge, and Christmas as well, are tied in with being cozy and comfortable.

Warm and comfortable blankets and pillows are ideal for scattering over seats and couches. Twist-up in a cover to sit in front of the TV on nights. Twist-up before the fireplace with a good book, enveloped by a warm, comfortable blanket.

Make your home look comfortable and welcoming to other people. Turn down the lights, light candles, give extraordinary food and drink.

Your house is the main spot for Hygge, so make it

warm, comfortable, and welcoming.

5. Do Cozy Activities

Cozy activities that you do alone, or with friends, are ideal for Christmas Hygge. There are such a large number of extraordinary comfortable exercises to do at Christmas time, alone or with others.

Welcome friends over and play board games before a roaring fire. Drink thought about wine and ate Christmas treats!

Comfortable up in a warm blanket and watch Christmas movies on your couch. Lay on your couch, hung with a cover, and read an incredible book!

Preparing is an extraordinarily comfortable movement, as are DIY crafts and projects.

Christmas exercises, for example, working out your Christmas cards and wrapping gifts, are acceptable comfortable Hygge exercises. Light candles, switch on Christmas music and work out the entirety of your cards for loved ones. Wrap and label your gifts and appreciate the occasion.

6. Play some Music

Christmas music truly fits Hygge. Relaxing Christmas tunes, for example, Frank Sinatra and Bing Crosby, played out of sight, will truly add to that warm, comfortable Hygge Christmas feeling!

7. Wear Cozy Clothes

The clothes you wear are so imperative to feeling comfortable, warm, and content.

It is alright to wear your night robe the entire day if you need to while laying on the couch reading a book or watching a film!

Wear warm garments (however not smothering), agreeable, and that vibe great. Fleece sweaters, warm knitted socks, PJs, and workout pants are all alright!

Finding satisfaction busy working – the "Hygge Way."

Nick Marks, a specialist on health, states: "Individuals who are happier at work are more profitable, increasingly connected with, more imaginative, and have better concentration."

Being happy grinding away is quintessential as we will,

in general, spend the better piece of our lives in the workplace.

This is the specific motivation behind why one should look for a calling that is certain to fulfill in the long-term.

You may be asking why we're mentioning this. Indeed, it turns out to work fulfillment has a great deal to do with the Scandinavian lifestyle and the hygge itself. And, this goes a long way past having some hygge-Esque plan components in your beginning up space.

Something beyond an insignificant plan thing, it's tied in with building up close to home space, having a sense of security, and motivated in the professional environment.

It is anything but an incident that the nations with hygge ingrained in their national DNA are also the ones with the absolute most liberal attitudes towards work plans.

Giving workers adequate measures of individual time and offering adaptability like this for increased profitability, Scandinavians, without a doubt, realize how to use hygge standards to the benefit of the enterprise.

Styling a hygge-Esque office

Leading – get the "right look."

Of course, we slammed the possibility of hygge being a shallow looks-just thing. And it truly isn't. The appearance does make a difference, as it assists with attaining the correct mentality.

Pick the correct shades

With regards to altering your office by hygge standards, it's about light tones – whites compared with beige and rosewood colors. Consolidating natural and mechanical, just as provincial and current moderate feel, is another quality that is quintessential to a genuine hygge experience.

By and by, this recommends the utilization of recovered wood, revamped furniture, and rough sawn elements. In certain respects, you may easily mistake hygge inside with natural stylistic layout style as both offer numerous comparative characteristics, depending heavily on clever mixes of natural and mechanical plan components.

The two styles, as often as possible, acquire components from one another and may even be utilized conversely or with regards to one another.

Keeping it warm with delicious beverages

If you love tea, espresso, or hot cocoa with some whipped cream and crushed spearmint candy sprinkled on top, at that point, you'll appreciate this part of hygge.

It's an obvious fact that an XXL-size mug with any of the referenced refreshments is a typical quality overall hygge-related imagery. The pattern has additionally found its way into the cutting edge office space.

Regardless of whether it's a central corporate command or a cooperating spot, bothering your path to the more elite classes isn't believable without a particular wooden table and a fuming cup of coffee resting on it.

Have some yummy snacks in your desk drawer

Where there's a cup of tasty drinks, will undoubtedly be a bowl of complementing snacks. Trust us, these simple, maybe even trite nuances make a major piece of a big motivator for hygge. Regardless of whether its home-made macaroons or a chocolate bar, having a delicious treat in an arm's span is the sort of a simple pleasure that makes the hygge magic work.

If you've at any point read one of the numerous hygge definitions, there's a once in a lifetime opportunity you saw a recurring pattern – the way of thinking firmly advocates being available.

Practically speaking, this means capitalizing on small-time delights. Read a book, record your thinking, thoughts, and keep an individual diary. Take frequent walks, change to bicycle as your essential methods for transportation.

Being in contact with nature around all of you, the while relaxing in your little world, are the foundations of care – definitive state of mind with regards to both understanding and getting a charge out of hygge.

Keep it innovative and individual

One of the most disregarded characteristics of hygge is the way that it opens space for immense creativity. Although certain tropes are basic to all hygge-motivated interiors, it doesn't mean you ought to blindly mirror the given an example without even the slightest bit of character. In short – there's no compelling reason to repeat an IKEA stock room look.

As such, explore, allow yourself little deviations from the subject, and, above everything, hush up about it genuine.

Motivational quotes or some other symbolism you

partner with achievements will be an invite expansion to your office space.

For a more close to home interpretation of the subject, you should seriously mull over a lot of Polaroid photographs showed on a cork wall or pegged to a wire that extends over the entire office space. Then again, you should use chalkboard walls to design and overhaul your office space as per your state of mind.

Let the nature inside your office space

Utilize plants. The greater the amount of them, the better. Aside from being a pure visual treat and easily supplementing your office inside, plants give normal methods for filtering the air around you and combat environment-induced stress.

Music saves lives

Another fundamental piece of Hygge theory is an audial delight.

Great music is attempted and tried the device for those experiencing difficulty keeping up their core interest. Improving one's work process and filling in as a good stress-reliever, carefully chosen music, will give a calming score to your day.

Our recommendation – this specially curated Spotify playlist, featuring tracks that will guarantee pleasant vibes without making you feel too comfortable to deliver your assignments.

Warm light

This one is simple – since Hygge is generally about feeling warm and comfortable inside and outside, it just bodes well to go through warm tones to light your office. Aside from the standard lighting that you should use for proficient duties, you can make an extraordinary state of mind by utilizing scented candles and string lights.

Go the "Scandi Way"

Presently, we feel compelled to pressure this one as much as possible. However, mimicking Nordic gratefulness for light and spacious insides is the correct approach in case you're seeking after the reading material hygge look.

With simplicity, utility, and magnificence at the center, Scandinavian houses/condos have a pure style that focuses on clean lines, warmth, and elegance. Practically speaking, this implies a ton of whites and hearty muted tones.

While floors ought to ideally be wooden, couches and easy chairs are frequently decorated with throw pillows and snuggly covers. Another significant thing to remember – try to dial back on accessories. Packed structure with lots of conspicuous tones is the total inverse of the great hygge look.

Some extra rules

Surrender to little yet rewarding pleasures

Try not to go excessively hard on yourself and remember that life's excellence is to be looked for in the little things. As such – don't deny yourself of the seemingly insignificant details that calm your soul.

Had a long and hard day at work – have that one glass of red wine. Had a good exercise at the rec center – allow yourself that one bit of chocolate. Try not to deny yourself of the seemingly insignificant details that soothe your soul.

Have a tech-detox in any event once in seven days

Presently, this may be a significant request to our tech-accustomed age, yet a day-long tech chaste is known to take care of no doubt.

This, in any case, doesn't mean total isolation and a sudden communication breakdown among you and your people. An incredible opposite – welcome them to your place and appreciate a genuine, eye-to-eye discussion with them. Nothing superior to restricting your online presence and trading it for a night of shared talks and laughter.

CHAPTER 5

HOW TO EMBRACE HYGGE IN THE WORKPLACE

1. Make your work area your own

Hygge is tied in with getting a charge out of the environment around you and changing individual spaces into little havens which allow us to sink into them at any minute.

In that capacity, Søderberg proposes that we customize our workplaces, however much as could be expected, emphasizing things which allow us to 'escape' the daily grind of the regular and set aside some effort to delight in the minor minutes that make you grin and inspire the soul.

"Bringing photographs, clippings, a most loved mug from home or a fun comic is an extraordinary method to add character to our workspace," she says. "Numerous work environments are structured in a very practical and streamlined way; however, to get some hygge, it assists with including character."

2. Bring the outdoors in with you

Hygge doesn't simply apply to comfortable indoor homes; we can also generate feelings of hygge by heading outside for a long walk, rummaging for regular berries, and appreciating the natural air against our skin.

Søderberg calls attention to that having a plant to take care of can assist with reproducing those happy vibes we get from being outside, including that they can have a surprisingly powerful impact on your mood at work.

"My closet came up short on a little life, so I carried a few plants to give it a little sparkle," she lets us know. "I was motivated by inside plan master, Christina b. Kjeldsen, who proposes gathering a few plants, so you have a beautiful green corner to lay your eyes on.

"I brought a little, vivid and cheap oxalis and a little cactus with a lovely purple flower. They don't require a lot of care; however, they are brilliant and inviting. At the point when I come to work and begin dressing up and doing my makeup, I generally give the oxalis a little water, and it has become a hyggelig part of my daily practice before the show."

3. Benefit as much as possible from your lunchtimes

Try not to spend your lunch break sitting at your work area; wrap up warm and head outside to get some food, get a few things done, take a walk, or snatch a book and locate a quiet spot to read.

4. Adjust your office lighting

"I need great light while doing my cosmetics, so the closet reflect has bulbs around it. But, I also have a good reading light on the table, where I can sit reading my content," clarifies Søderberg.

"To make the lighting hyggelig, it is crucial to have a few lights with warm, somewhat orange, light around the room, making pools of light - little light caves where you can inundate immerse in your work.

"A good working light on the table would be where the shade covers the bulb, so the light falls directly onto the papers and work on the table, and doesn't shine directly into the eyes, which is neither useful for the focus and nor for the hygge."

If your office allows candles, it's additionally worth putting resources into a decent scented one.

"There is a great deal of hygge in flame light, so I have carried one with me to the auditorium for when I plunk down to prepare," says Søderberg.

"The activity of lighting it makes me mindful existing apart from everything else in a unique manner. It is an approach to share myself a sign that now the time has come to work in a hyggelig way."

5. Keep extra layers at work

As the colder months settle in, and as fights over the conditioning rage on, it's a smart thought to store some comfortable layers at work. This could be a cashmere jumper, a vivid scarf, an extra pair of socks (ideal for when the rain soaks your shoes directly through), or a cuddly cape cardigan – the nearest we can find a good pace into a blanket busy working.

6. Take a break

Putting forth a conscious effort to stop work for a minute, regardless of whether it's simply to make some tea in your unique mug, is essential to a hyggelig work environment. Keep a reserve of your most loved teabags in your cabinet, and ensure you use them.

7. Try not to sit in one spot

You don't need to remain chained to your work area throughout the day; Søderberg proposes being inventive with your workspace, so you move around for various exercises.

She explains: "The most hyggelig thing in my closet are the two couches toward the finish of the room that consistently welcome me to sit down and get comfortable while I read content without anyone else, or while practicing lines and talking about the content together with one of my associates.

"If your office has space for a couch or sofa, easy chair to dedicate yourself completely to, it very well may be a good option in contrast to sitting still at the table.

"It regularly makes the working day more hyggelig to understand messages, compose a plan for the day or call somebody while drinking some tea on the couch."

8. Make an office playlist

Tuning in to music shields things from feeling excessively cruel or calm; regardless of whether it's having everybody in the workplace concur on a radio broadcast, or flying on your earphones and tuning into something soothing, music is vital to a good hyggelig condition.

Attempt to pick songs that evoke feelings of warmth and closeness at every possible opportunity. A few suggestions incorporate Mumford and Sons' I Will Wait, Radiohead's everything in Its Right Place, or Touch the Sky by Julie Fowlis.

9. Focus on finding happiness at work

Hygge is as of now in our lexicons, yet it worth adding another carefully Danish word to your collection, arbejdsglæde. Arbejde means work and glade means happiness, so arbejdsglæde is "satisfaction at working."

In Denmark and other Scandinavian nations, work isn't only an approach to get paid – they completely hope to have a significant level of employment fulfillment and happiness, as well.

This can be achieved through adaptable working hours, or incredible employee advantages, or normal preparing (Danes love to drive themselves to learn new things), or through managers giving less immediate requests (they favor laborers to feel enabled).

In any case, if this isn't available at your office, you can generally locate your arbejdsglæde by commending the people around you, by performing irregular demonstrations of work environment kindness, by taking a normal portion of personal time every day, and by keeping natural product around your work area to snack for the day.

10. Bond with your colleagues

"Hygge is the feeling of being seen and perceived - and to be surrounded by the natural and well-known," says Søderberg – which is the reason manufacturing associations with your partners is so significant. Regardless of whether it's a contribution to make everybody some tea, getting some information about their day, organizing customary one-on-one feedback sessions, or proposing unordinary meeting areas (try a walk-and-talk, or take everybody outside for a hold up).

You could also organize an enjoyable activity for all of you to attempt together, for example, visiting a local café together at noon or taking drinks at the bar after work.

"Snatch a brew after work, let the covers fall, and hygge together," proposes Søderberg.

Anyway, your enjoyment doesn't need to be restricted to outside the workplace; you could also sort out a sweepstake, take an hour out to play a group table game, try meditation meetings at noon, or plunk down together for a comfortable visit over a cuppa and a few biscuits.

You could even sort out a tasty food rota, with individuals taking it in goes to get handcrafted cakes or soup for the workplace.

Whatever you choose, it merits diving in; all things considered, there is nothing more hyggelig than setting aside a few minutes for people.

3 Ways in Which You Can Adopt the Principles of Hygge in the Workplace

You can find a way to empower the comfort and feeling of satisfaction regularly connected with hygge. At work, this means making the correct culture, offering keen advantages, and guaranteeing that employees experience little moments of happiness and satisfaction as a major aspect of their everyday workday. Here are three different ways you can take motivation from hygge and rethink your work culture.

1. Open up communication across the organization

At the point when done right, hygge at work should

leave each worker feeling happy and empowered. This can't happen if you have a rigid authoritative pecking order with limited communication between the diverse saw positions. Rather, it is prudent to follow an in formalized structure where each employee is treated as an individual and a similarly significant supporter of business results.

By opening the lines of effective communication in the work environment across senior leaders, specialty unit heads, officials, and assistants – while publicly supporting thoughts from the whole workforce – you can make a culture of majority rule government and strengthen. It's nothing unexpected; at that point that an open office design that energizes quick casual talks is among the fundamental precepts of hygge at work.

2. Make employee wellness central to your benefits package

Again and again, bosses limit their advantages to the mandatory time-offs and clinical strategies as ordered by the government. Monetary compensation should make up for the lack of any worth expansion to employee well-being.

This lack of focus on worker well-being makes a work environment where employees routinely battle with different individual and expert difficulties. For instance, student debt and psychological well-being issues could be affecting employee happiness. Also, these are issues that businesses can address through explicit measures.

Offering worker-driven advantages like a sound cafeteria, educational cost repayment, emotional well-being support, financial well-being, arrangements for childcare, and other such advantages, can go far towards enabling hygge at work.

3. Energize sustainable relationships between employees and their environment

Keep in mind, at work, hygge is firmly connected with how workers respond to and communicate with their environment. By moving in the direction of maintainability, you can fabricate a sound connection among employees and their surroundings, making them bound to experience "hygge" at work.

Keeping away from paper-based procedures, decreasing the requirement for long drives by offering adaptability and remote work choices, and giving reasonable food options are a portion of the key advances you can take to make a culture of supportability in the working environment.

Hygge in the Early Years

Meik Wiking from the Happiness Research Institute in Copenhagen (and the writer of The Little Book of Hygge) accepts that 10 distinct elements must be viewed as while embracing a hygge way of life:

Atmosphere – making a quiet vibe.

Nearness – not being on your telephone and living at the time.

Delight – life ought to be fun, pleasant, and bring great happiness.

Fairness – nobody is better than any other person.

Fellowship – spend time with people you care about and those that make you grin.

Appreciation – set aside an effort to consider what you're thankful for.

Harmony – life isn't an opposition.

Truce – there's no requirement for arguments.

Comfort – relax, wear fluffy socks, and be comfortable.

Asylum – your house is significant.

Accepting this as a beginning stage, I accept there are numerous simple, reasonable ways that we can bring the hygge theory into our arrangement. Here is a selection you may jump at the chance to try:

- Try swapping your brutal strip lighting for lights, pixie lights, and LED candles.

- Create comfortable resting niches in which kids and adults can share a book.

- Add warm surfaces to your condition, for instance, sheepskin carpets, soft pads, and weaved tosses.

- Bring nature into your arrangement at each chance.

- Share extraordinary memories you've had all together by printing them out and placing them in photo frames.

- Create little places to talk and be as one. Add some intriguing items to them to empower conversation.

- Try to clean up your learning surroundings to cause them to feel like more settled spaces.

- Take motivation from Scandi inside the plan and go for more neutral colors like whites and grays.

Case study: Daisy Chain Nursery

The group at Daisy Chain Nursery has been working hard to bring the hygge feeling into their condition.

A quieting impact

At the point when the choice was made to change the nursery's approach, the group began by adjusting the furnishings and quieting the coloring to make a more characteristic feel, and quickly saw an adjustment in the behavior of the two-year-old kids, just as the kids who have special educational needs.

The youngsters appeared to be much more settled, and the situations, by and large, appeared to be less frantic, as kids were locked in by the toys and the exercises on offer as opposed to being overstimulated by their environment.

The group additionally saw that the youngsters were settling in much quicker, as a ton of the decorative objects included were things they would almost certainly discover in their own homes, while the common colors were helping them feel more comfortable.

Room by room

The nursery started the procedure in the infant room and began by adjusting how work was shown and buying new floor rugs and fresh equipment to make the room look more natural.

Plants were acquainted with the earth and normal colored materials and warm white lighting consolidated to give the room a comfortable vibe that you felt when you walked in.

The group utilized a lot of soft decorations and included a teepee loaded up with wooden and characteristic free parts for exploration.

They, at that point, proceeded onward to the two-year-old arrangement. There was some worry now about how specialists would fit the important taking into the home-from-home methodology; anyway, it was quickly established that the procedure is more focused around how you show the things you have just as the effect moving away from 'toys' can have on the youngsters.

The group manufactured a huge sandpit and made it into a natural communication-friendly space, and this has bigly affected the youngsters as they have a safe space to proceed to play where they can utilize their entire bodies.

More natural resources were added to the preschool room. Initially, a large portion of the current decorations was held; however, the group is right now during the time spent adjusting both furnishings and assets to make a significantly cozier area following the acquisition of the business' subsequent setting…

Ongoing development

From the beginning, the group tried to change their new setting following their home-from-home methodology. The new nursery is in an old Victorian house, and 'hygge' fit the character of the structure significantly more, so they had the option to revamp the areas and make them comfortable and normal rapidly.

Once more, this immediately affected the kids, quieting their behavior, and helping experts see how to utilize the continuous provision as a learning asset.

The preschool room inside the new setting is extraordinary compared to other normal learning situations the group has made up until now, illustrating how the procedure is consistently advancing.

A change will benefit you

Utilizing a hygge approach, there are some basic changes we would all be able to cause to our arrangement to assist us with feeling quieter and appreciate each day. Consider what your youngsters and group need, and if you give it a go, make certain to set aside a few minutes for ordinary reflections on how the change is going and the effect it's having on every one of those included.

CHAPTER # 6

HOW TO PRACTICE HYGGE FOR WINTER SELF-CARE

Since winter is here, it's the ideal opportunity for you to comfortable up with your projectile diary (and a hot cup of cocoa!) for a much-needed slow-down after the Christmas and New Year's hurricane.

I've been reading The Little Book of Hygge (articulate Hoo-ga) for thoughts on the best way to rehearse hygge for winter self-care.

In Danish, hygge means comfort, peace, and health — this sweet, outlined guide provokes us to "get deliberately comfortable."

Making a bullet journal collection page for hygge thoughts will make it simpler to fit them into even the most tightly packed schedules.

Why Practice Hygge for Winter Self-Care?

Danes reliably rate as probably the happiest people on Earth, in show disdain toward those well-known long, cool, dull winters.

You don't should be from Denmark to need hygge minutes, and with these winter self-care tips, you can also feel cozier during a blizzard or any winter climate condition.

The lack of daylight and short sunshine hours are discouraging for a large number of us, and seasonal affective disorder (SAD) is normal.

Megan, over at her blog, Page Flutter, has some awesome thoughts regarding how to add hygge exercises to your shot diary. Look at it!

Have Candlelight in Your Home

In case you live in Denmark, at that point, you will once in a while, find scented candles in plain view in a home; however, you will find unscented lit candles.

Most Danish individuals have a great deal of plain white candles all through the house (or even the workplace!), and they light the candles to make a comfortable mood.

The unscented candles are lit for the day and are in each room.

Search for plain white candles at a local store, and spot

the things in candle-holders all through your home to make a cozy atmosphere.

Cook Your Favorite Comfort Foods

In the winter, you can overcome the feeling of darkness by cooking your preferred comfort foods.

You should have a warm bowl of macaroni and cheese, or you may favor pureed potatoes with fried chicken.

To expand the emotions of comfort, you could welcome your friends to your home to appreciate a potluck buffet of comfort foods.

You can also host a cooking get-together to figure out how to set up the most well-known comfort foods from Denmark.

Make a Quiet Oasis inside Your Home

You ought to also have a calm oasis spring inside your home where you can rest and relax following a tough day at work.

This unique area may be a seat by the window that is loaded up with soft pillows and a warm cover so you can peruse your preferred book.

Or on the other hand, you may have a calm area in your

lounge or room that causes you to feel peaceful and cozy.

Visit a Nearby Cafe

On the ends of the week, you ought to have a most loved cafe to visit with your friends where you can sit for a considerable length of time looking at nothing while at the same time drinking cups of coffee and eating delicious desserts.

While spending time with your friends, you may have a serious feeling of happiness or comfort that is indefinable, making it a hygge minute.

Appreciate a Favorite Hobby in the winter

If you don't possess energy for a diversion during different seasons, at that point, you will have time in the winter.

Choose a hobby that you can appreciate at home or with your friends. You should figure out how to weave in the winter, and this is a hobby that you can take with you to a friend's home.

Extra comfortable minutes in the winter can remember lighting a fire for a chimney before relaxing before it to tune in to music.

Or then again, you can have a warm air pocket shower before applying moisturizer on your dry skin.

Make Cozy Moments in the Winter with a Home Spa Day

Going through a day at a spa leaves you feeling relaxed, refreshed, and all-around mind-boggling. In any case, they additionally come with a price tag that puts them distant on a day by day or even weekly basis.

It is conceivable to appreciate a spa day without the costly price tag, however: a spa day at home!

Here are a few different ways you can reproduce the spa day involvement with the home.

Light Scented Aromatherapy Candles

Perhaps the best advantage of an at-home spa day is that you can utilize your preferred scented candles to customize the experience truly.

(Danes use unscented candles, yet we can go wild with fragrance!)

Get a few of your preferred scented candles in lavender, lemongrass, orange, tangerine, vanilla — are largely yummy aromas, particularly when made with 100% soy wax and fundamental oils.

Light them and appreciate the soothing fragrance, soft light, and gentle warmth they give.

Load up on Supplies

Hit up the medication store, large box store, or general store and load up on all the things you requirement for a spa day.

I am pampering supplies: face veils, rich salves, lavish cleanser and conditioner, nail treatment, and pedicure things (counting a stunning color of polish).

Remember fragrant oil or shower salts so you can thrive in a nice, warm tub.

In the produce walkway, get a few cucumbers or natural products to flavor your water.

Remember the Music

Climate and mood are everything!

So for a spa-like experience, go for some delicate, mitigating old style, or maybe some Enya.

If you have a full-house speaker framework, this would be perfect so that you can hear your music all through the house.

Something else, make a custom playlist on your telephone, associate it to a Bluetooth speaker, and move it around with you.

Take as much time as is needed

In today's busy world, we tend to hurry through everything. In any event, when there's a three day weekend, tasks, or in any event, reading a book will, in general, be hurried through.

For this to be a genuine spa day, you have to kick back and take as much time as is needed. Relish each understanding of the day.

Try not to be enticed to perform multiple tasks and apply the face cover while you absorb the tub.

Leave every individual experience alone, it's own, and focuses on all the scents, sights, sounds, surfaces, and feelings each brings.

Get rid of all Distractions

Ensure you won't be upset. Mood killer your telephone, your tablet, and your PC. Turn the ringer down on your landline, and consider disconnecting the doorbell.

Ignore the outside world and focus on your spa day. Allow yourself to relax and revive by offering yourself a total break from day by day life.

Treat yourself and appreciate the isolation and tranquility of being in the solace of your own home as you spoil yourself.

Lastly, the Bullet Journal!

Winter is the ideal time to cuddle up with a note pad and pen and make fabulous designs, collections, or page spreads.

You may be in a hurry a large portion of summer, yet when the climate turns cold, and you're comfortable inside, you might be motivated to slow off and doodle, coloring, sketch, or draw complex trackers and different plans.

For hygge doodle thoughts, look at the plans you see on the picture below. They were made by art, Koko, who lives in Denmark with her significant other and youthful child.

Winter Self-Care Activities for Your Bullet Journal (Includes hygge, and other self-care thoughts for winter.)

Winter comes around consistently, reminding us to withdraw inside. As we cuddle underneath our covers to get away from the chilly, we ought to make sure to support our bodies and minds.

Set aside the effort to do the things you appreciate, things that will lift your spirits regardless of what the climate might be.

At the point when we do these things, we will be well on our way to achieving the ideal parity of winter self-care.

Hygge-Inspired Traveler

In the course of the most recent couple of years, it appears that each industry – from design and travel to form and nourishment – has excitedly gotten on board with the hygge fleeting trend. News sources extending from The New York Times and Forbes to The Food Network and Travel and Leisure have all touted the uplifting idea, which is as yet warming up today. Soon after the New Year, US News and World Report ran a story on "The Coziest Cities in America" (I'm lucky to reside in one!), and a month ago, Visit Cook County Minnesota facilitated its third yearly hygge celebration.

The Hygge Palate – Eateries and Culinary Classes

Restaurants, coffee houses, lounges, pubs, and bakeries that offer comfort menu choices would all be able to be considered hygge. Think hot drinks soak tea, smooth hot cocoa, or thought about wine (referred to as Glögg in Scandinavia). The Little Book of Hygge by Miek Wiking emphasizes that something evil is an essential part of the custom, along these lines, enjoying cake or a cake during movement is a during travel is a must. Togetherness is also part of the subject. Here, culinary visits and cooking classes for little gatherings can become possibly the most important factor. For instance, a visit to a rancher's market that closes with the members planning moderately cooked dishes, for example, stews or meals, can lead the casual association among voyagers and energy about the nourishment.

Interfacing with Nature – Outdoor Activities or Organic Interior Elements

The Hygge Life includes that being surrounded by nature enables people to cut their watchman down and value a specific simplicity. Here, it's time to give up yourself to be available. Journeys to blooming gardens, grand parks, vessel travels, or beautiful mountain climbs all allow guests to take in hygge. The idea also incorporates bringing nature inside. Cause to notice housing that bestows nature into the stylistic theme, regardless of whether wooden cabinets or seats, extraordinary plants, or Christmas trees during the special seasons.

Lighting – Lamps, Fires or Rays of Sunshine

Rooms equipped with delicate low lighting, a crackling fireplace, or soothing lit candles (non-scented) all assistance make what is referred to as an enthusiastic comfort. Especially during the long periods of shorter daylight, these aides gently light up inside the environment. During the hotter season, less emphasis is on candles, however, exploiting the immediate characteristic daylight in the outside. Itineraries that incorporate waterfront exercises, biking, picnics, or eating in the open air under the open sky all show spring or mid-year hygge.

Soft Textures – Attire and Accessories

From clothing to furniture décor, easygoing and agreeable is vital. For cooler temperatures, urge visitors to bring along wool socks, layers of soft garments, and scarves. For open-air exercises, it's tied in with packaging up in snuggly fabrics. Consider organizing a comfortable scene where visitors can twist up in fluffy throw blankets, soft pillows, cushions, or sheepskin mats. Keep the colors normal with tints of whites, grays, or light pinks.

Tokens of Gratitude – Hygge-Inspired Gifts

Welcome guests with a duplicate of the hygge manifesto and treat them to a diary for reflections on their experiences along their trip. Upon flight, send them away with nearby things to grant hygge into their home – a flame, tea or homemade jam, or a carved crystal from the earth.

Careful discipline brings about promising results – Your Turn at Hygge

Sort out an office or at-home party to try the Danish fine art and observe how it causes everybody to feel. Have visitors join to bring hygge-themed food pot-luck style (a potato bar, flame-broiled cheese sandwiches, reflected on wine and chocolate fondue were hits at Break the Ice Media!). Illuminate everybody to dress in like manner and thoughtfully place candles, plants, and soft covers and pillows around the room.

The experience makes for a wonderful break that will motivate your group to slow down (phones are not allowed), fraternize over consoling treats and support feeling thankful for where you at this moment.

YOU DON'T WANT HYGGE. YOU WANT SOCIAL DEMOCRACY.

It's the special seasons, and you long to be comfortable.

You need to twist up in a plush armchair next by a snapping fire. You need the gentlest of covers and wooliest of sweaters. You need to eat up grandmother's walnut fudge, get tipsy on eggnog with your cousins, and watch Miracle on 34th Street — mother's top pick — for the thirty-fourth time. Or then again perhaps neither Christmas nor family social occasions are your things, yet you like tasting hot drinks and playing board games with a couple of dear friends while outside the snow falls and the lights twinkle.

However, you can't have it, since you couldn't spring on a plane ticket. Or on the other hand, family members are visiting the area, yet times are tight, and it appeared to be unreliable to leave behind the Christmas extra time pay. Possibly everything incidentally became all-good; however, you can't relax. You're looking at your inbox, on edge about the work that is not completing. You're a minute ago shopping, keeping a tight budget, thinking Scrooge had some reasonable focuses. Or on the other hand, you're hiding in your childhood bedroom, marathon watching TV and looking over social media because an uncommon break from the weights of everyday life feels more like an event to day-dream than to celebrate and be cheerful.

In any case, you feel bad because you realize that somebody someplace is cooking chestnuts on an open fire, and you're passing up a major opportunity.

The Danes have a word for the thing you desperately need yet can't show: hygge.

The word isn't anything but difficult to translate. It originates from a Norwegian word that signifies "well-being," yet the contemporary Danish definition is more expansive than that.

In The Little Book of Hygge: Danish Secrets to Happy Living, writer Meik Wiking states, "Hygge is about an environment and an experience, instead of about things. It's tied in with being with our loved ones. A feeling of home. A feeling that we are safe, that we are protected from the world and allowed to let our gatekeeper to down."

You can have hygge whenever, however, Danes firmly partner it with Christmas, the most hyggelig season. When asked what things they partner most with hygge,

Danes replied, arranged by significance: hot drinks, candles, chimneys, Christmas, board games, music, occasion, desserts and cake, cooking, and books. Seven out of ten Danes state hygge is best experienced at home, and they even have a word for it — hjemmehygge, or home hygge.

But, Wiking stresses that while hygge has strong, stylish properties, it's more than the whole of its parts. You don't simply observe it, you feel it.

"Hygge means that you believe the ones you are with and where you are," he expresses, "that you have extended your usual range of familiarity to incorporate others, and you believe you can be yourself around others." something contrary to hygge is alienation.

It's no coincidence event that this idea is both local to and universally understood in a similar nation that consistently dominates the World Happiness Report and other yearly reviews of general satisfaction. On rare events, when another country outperforms Denmark, that country is constantly a Scandinavian neighbor.

What makes individuals in these countries happier than all of us is quite basic. Danes and their neighbors have greater access to the structure squares of satisfaction: time, organization, and security.

Scandinavians don't have these things since they esteem them more, or for social reasons that are intrinsic, irreplaceable, and past our range—individuals everywhere throughout the world worth time, organization, and security. What Scandinavians do have is a political-economic arrangement of action that better encourages the ordinary expression of those qualities. That course of action is social democracy.

THE POLITICS OF HYGGE

Denmark is certifiably not a socialist country, however like its neighbor Sweden, it came near the collectivizing industry during the 1970s. That effort was driven by "associations, well-known developments, and left parties," compose Andreas Møller Mulvad and Rune Møller Stahl in Jacobin. "It was these mass powers — not benevolent elites, carefully weighing the options before settling on an enlightened mix of free enterprise and socialism — who were the planners and driving force behind the Nordic model. They are the ones answerable for making the Nordic nations among the happiest and most democratic in the world."

A strong capitalist offensive prevented this Scandinavian coalition from understanding the change to communism, and the heritage of their efforts is a fragile trade-off. The private area perseveres, however, imposes both dynamic and high no matter how you look at it. The nation burns through 55 percent of its all-out GDP freely, making it the third-most elevated government high-roller per capital on the world. In the meantime, the power of employers is, in part, checked by strong associations, to which 66% of Danes have a place.

This redistributive course of action altogether lessens the class stratification that originates from free enterprise. Subsequently, Denmark has probably the highest degrees of financial equality in the world.

The entirety of that open spending goes to financing a strong welfare state. Everyone pays in, and everyone receives the benefits. This libertarian, humane, and solidarity model permits the qualities related to hygge to prosper. It additionally gives individuals more chances to follow up on them.

In Denmark, human services are free at the point of service. The same goes for instruction, entirely through school and even graduate school. 20% of the Danish housing stock is social lodging, managed, and financially supported by the state, however, claimed in like manner by occupants, and written in the "custom of inhabitants' cooperation and self-service." Denmark offers year-since quite a while ago paid parental leave, and ensures widespread kid care for all youngsters starting the minute that leaves closes, when the child is one year old.

So also, due in enormous part to the past and present quality of associations, Denmark has worker-friendly labor laws and benchmarks which make for a more harmonious work-life balance. Danes get five weeks' paid get-away, in addition to an extra nine public holidays. In contrast to the United States, Denmark has a national paid debilitated leave approach. Denmark additionally has generous unemployment benefits and a compensation endowment program for individuals who need to work at the same time, for reasons beyond their ability to do anything about, need more flexible arrangements.

The ordinary workweek in Denmark is set at thirty-seven hours, and individuals will, in general, stick to it. Just 2 percent of Danes report working extended periods. In a study of OECD nations, Denmark ranked fourth for individuals investing the most energy dedicated to recreation and personal care. (The US positioned thirtieth.)

The entirety of this profoundly affects people's capacity to experience delight, trust, comfort, closeness, significant serenity — and, the composite of these things, hygge.

For a certain something, there are just such huge numbers of hours in a day. Also, there are a few exercises that satisfy us, and some that make us unhappy.

The Princeton Affect and Time Survey found that the exercises that make us happiest incorporate playing with kids, tuning in to music, being outside, going to parties, working out, spending time with friends, and spending time with pets. (These are also the exercises that Danes partner with hygge.) The ones that satisfy us least incorporate paid work, local work, home support and fixes, getting things done, personal medical care, and dealing with financial responsibilities.

Everybody needs to do exercises in the troubled class to keep their affairs in control. However, it bodes well that if you take a portion of those duties off individuals' plates and plan the economy to give them more opportunity to do exercises in the happy category, they will be more content and lead additionally enhancing lives.

Many common laborers Americans don't possess a lot of energy for exercises in the cheerful class since they maintain various sources of income or extended periods and need to maintain a family unit in order without much assistance. A lot more are worried about the possibility that if they remove time from their stressful obligations, they will ignore something significant and fall behind, and there will be no social well-being net to get them —pervasive anxiety that creeps up up the class hierarchy. This breeds alienation, not closeness.

Also, working individuals in highly capitalist countries, where financial life is described by cutthroat competition and the discipline for losing the opposition, is destitution, will, in general, create hostile relationships with each other, which isn't very hyggelig.

The social-majority rule model is predicated rather on solidarity: my neighbor and I both make good on charges with the goal that we can both have an elevated expectation of living. We care for one another on the guarantee that we will each be thought about. By cooperating rather than against one another, we both get what we need. Widespread social projects like those that make up the Scandinavian government assistance states are accordingly engines of solidarity, putting forth for individuals that their neighbor isn't a rival or an obstacle, yet a partner in building and looking after society.

By setting individuals in opposition to one another, the

neoliberal capitalist enterprise advances doubt and hostility. This much of the time maps onto social divisions and shows as prejudice, sexism, xenophobia, etc. However, it additionally just makes individuals protected and single as a rule. Individuals who live in social majority rule governments are a long way from immune to prejudice or misanthropy, however the social minimal stays bound to advance benevolence, trust, and altruism among individuals than neoliberal private enterprise — and without a doubt, the Danes are probably the most trusting people in the world, of friends and outsiders the same.

One of these political-economic arrangements strengthens individuals' association with the essentials of happiness, and hygge — time, organization, and security — while the different cuts off it. The bounty or shortage of these essentials shapes the material basis of aggregate public activity.

How to Have a Hygge Staycation

Odds are, you've heard the word hygge (articulated HOO-ga) being tossed around starting late. For the unexposed, Hygge House gives an extraordinary definition: "Hygge is a Danish word that is a feeling or mood that comes [from] enjoying certifiable making common, consistently minutes more important, delightful or unique."

Hygge is absolutely what you think about it.

The word summons the comfort of a lodge in Scandinavia, light snow falling while you read your preferred book before a chimney. Hygge is about what you decided to do during the day, and how it benefits your general condition of quiet. It's a hard word to characterize because it is anything but a physical thing.

I spent time in Iceland, and it just felt unique. The light was softer, voices appeared to be quieted, and things moved a piece more slow by and large. It wasn't until another person informed me regarding the possibility of hygge that it clicked: the individuals I experienced were setting aside the effort to appreciate what they were doing, regardless of whether it was serving a beverage at a bar or offering coffee to a friend or family member.

Previously, I would call it "personal time." Taking one moment to detach from the nagging world of social media and telephone applications and appreciate the organization of another person—or only a couple of moments of quiet making tea all alone.

There are a lot of aides out there on the best way to more readily take advantage of hygge in your home; however, perhaps the most ideal approach to embrace the way of life is by immersing yourself in it during a staycation. The best part is, you don't need to make a lot of changes—you need to focus on doing things carefully and setting aside the best possible effort to appreciate them.

You're just several means from getting yourself a hygge staycation. Here's how I propose going about it:

Buy a New Candle

There is something in particular about flashing candlelight that truly sets the mood. Set up tea lights in the spots you visit most in your home or place a major flame in your room. Get yourself a present and select a light with numerous wicks in your favorite scent (hello, even staycations merit gifts).

Treat Yourself to a New Book

Reading is one of those interests that turns into the principal thing to fall to the wayside when faced with a busy schedule. Give yourself a whole evening and get that book you've been trying to complete, get a most loved story, or purchase a soft blanket you've for a long while been wanted to read. In case you have a fireplace, make a point to set yourself up before it with a glass of tea, or reflected on wine.

Plan a Weekend of Meals You've Always Wanted to Cook

Before you officially kick off your hygge staycation, plan out two days of dinners and bites that you need to get ready for yourself (or two or three friends!). Pull out the cookbooks or hit the Internet for motivation— Smitten Kitchen has a ton of simple plans loaded with soothing flavors. Try not to make this about eating healthy; make it about your favorite ingredients. You are on vacation.

At the point when you do get down to the cooking, truly set aside the effort to appreciate it. Put on your favorite album, set out the fixings, and have a great time. Hygge is a lot of care as it is in vogue.

Find a workable pace, to Make Tea or Coffee

On the principal day of your hygge-action, find a good pace sooner than your end of the week wake-up time and make your morning refreshment as opposed to getting it. Consider it a morning meditation, with a particularly flavorful result.

Go through 30 Minutes Journaling

While you're making the most of your coffee or tea, get

a diary and begin writing. You needn't bother with a brief—in case you're having issues beginning, beginning writing on what you did the day preceding.

At that point Go Back to Bed and Cover Yourself in Blankets

After you've done your journaling, head back to bed to watch a film, or lay buried in blankets (the greater, the better). Hygge is tied in with feeling comfortable, and there's nothing cozier than taking a snappy early in the day snooze as the light of the day streams into your home. Set aside some effort to tune in to your home as it sinks into the day. If it's pleasant out, open a window and tune in to the distinctive morning sounds happening outside.

Take a Long Bath

Avoid the shower and pick a bath. In case you're truly betting everything, prepare and purchase a scented shower bomb or soaking salts. Snatch that book you were reading and take in a story before the water gets too cold.

Welcome a Friend Over for a Glass of Wine—or Tea

Continuously or the third day, you might be feeling

somewhat exhausted in your hygge home. The best arrangement? Welcome a friend over for supper. Take a stab at cooking together, eating together, and simply sharing stories over a glass of post-supper tea or wine. Once more, the fireplace suggested.

Detach From All Electronics, Even If Just for an Afternoon

Perhaps the best thing about hygge is that it truly is tied in with making a comfortable space. If you don't need that space to incorporate steady telephone notices, turn it off. If the idea of separating for an entire day sends you into a fit of anxiety, try it for an hour or two.

Surprisingly better: Head into your neighborhood with no arrangement (or Google Maps), and go through the early evening time examining shops. End the day by picking another spot for supper.

Try Your Hand at Water-coloring

Causing things with your hands to can be incredibly therapeutic, if just for the update that creativity isn't simply something you see on a screen. Get a watercolor palette, a brush, blended media paper, and a cup with water, and find a workable pace. There's no set in stone with regards to painting.

If water-coloring isn't your thing, take a stab at instructing yourself to weave through YouTube videos or snatch a coloring book. Depending upon where you live, you could read a canvas or ceramics class, also. Anything that removes you from your conventional daily schedule.

Go for a Long Stroll in Nature

After having the opportunity to quiet yourself to the very center, head outside, and take in the spots you visit each day. Odds are you'll perceive new details when you set aside the effort to back off and digest your environment. Scandinavian countries have been named the happiest, and the measure of time they spent outside is thought to have something to do with that. Call up your favorite people, and take that hike.

CHAPTER # 7

HYGGE CONSPIRACY:

I nevitably and unexpectedly, Britain has been attacked by hygge. The Danish word, already obscure to everything except the most in-your-face Scandophiles, is presently the subject of an avalanche of books, many Identikit paper features, and endless department-store winter shows. Each story regarding the matter clarifies that the word opposes strict interpretation, before offering "comfort" as a functional guess – it's not actually that, yet rather, a feeling of quiet peace and the delight in basic joys, maybe lit up by the delicate flicker of candlelight.

Not the least of the mysteries of this craze, which you may also call a wildly overhyped pattern, is that just pronouncing it is practically outlandish for British tongues. The main notice of hygge in any content – where it sits so invitingly on the page, with its column of well-proportioned descenders – ordinarily comes with a phonetic guide. This is to keep readers from submitting the socially bad act of expressing "higgy" or "huggy" – or, more regrettable, "high." "Tone gah," "hoo-gah," "heurgh," and "hhyooguh" are among the approximations offered in the (in any event) nine books on hygge distributed this pre-winter. (The Sun, supportively, proposes it should rhyme with "cougar.")

The titles of these books, deliberately adjusted for site design improvement, are Hygge: The Danish Art of Happiness; The Little Book of Hygge: The Danish Way to Live Well; Hygge: A Celebration of Simple Pleasures, Living the Danish Way; The Cozy Life: Rediscover the Joy of Simple Things Through the Danish Concept of Hygge; Hygge: The Complete Guide to Embracing the Danish Concept of Cozy and Simple Living; The Art of Hygge: How to Bring Danish Coziness Into Your Life; How to Hygge: The Secrets of Nordic Living; The Book of Hygge: The Danish Art of Living Well; Keep Calm and Hygge: A Guide to the Danish Art of Simple and Cozy Living.

The hygge conspiracy – podcast

"It is the most striking distributing pattern I can recall, regarding the sheer number of titles distributed simultaneously," Caroline Sanderson, who expounds on true to life for the Bookseller magazine, let me know. Thus, unavoidably, there is also a tenth book – a spoof. Its distribution was reported just 29 days after the first of the straight books turned out. State Ja to Hygge: How to Find Your Special Cozy Place recommends that the significant word be pronounced "huhhpg-ghuhrr." This isn't the main event when the farce is difficult to recognize from the volumes it is spoofing.

Similarly as "chic" is what everybody thinks about the French, the word hygge should now be fastened, nearly by law, to any media story about Denmark or, without a doubt, anything remotely Scandinavian, regardless of whether the subject is garments, furniture, cookery, travel, or working hours. The features are generally silly. Get Hygge with It! Hungry For Hygge! Ten Reasons to Hygge … It Will Makes You Happier, Fitter, and Slimmer! Give Your Home a Hygge! There is even a New Statesman article titled The Hygge of Oasis: Why I Find This Band Strangely Comforting.

As indicated by this now huge famous writing, the formation of an environment of hygge is supported by glögg (thought about wine), meatballs, and cardamom buns. Certain exercises and entertainments, frequently including candles, woolens, or nature, are additionally said to promote feelings of hygge. One of the less modern books suggests projects for making "winter hitting" and a "mug cozy," the last to be designed from buttons, sequins, and an old sock. Its recommendation to take up the hyggelig action of cycling is joined by an inspirational statement from that apothegm of existential happiness, Sylvia Plath.

I have seen hygge used to sell cashmere cardigans, wine, backdrop, vegetarian shepherd's pie, sewing designs, a skincare run, small merry outfits for dachshunds, yoga withdraws and an occasion in a "shepherd's cabin" in Kent. The Royal and Derngate Theater in Northampton has even opened a Bar Hygge – specialty brew and open sandwiches a strength. "It's difficult to pinpoint a definition for the Danish word 'hygge,'" declares the site. "It sits somewhere close to warmth and cozy, comfort and fellowship, capitalizing on each minute, away from stresses. We needed to obtain a portion of that and carry it to Northampton."

Hygge has been recorded as a "word of the year" by both the Collins and Oxford word references – close by Brexit and Trumpism – in the lexicographers' yearly advertising exercise. Trembling of a hygge kickback, found in plays, for example, a Daily Mash piece titled Hygge Is Byllshytte, serve to emphasize its ubiquity. The Eurosceptic Daily Telegraph ran an article proposing that readers receive a "bracingly British" form of the pattern – brygge.

One morning in October, I walked around John Lewis' London leader store with Philippa Prinsloo, it's head of the plan: we ran our hands over fake-fur throws and heated water bottles, felt the nub of Scottish woolen covers, respected hyggelig silverware that supported sharing and simplicity. The subject of the home-ware shows was, she stated, "winter warmth. Ensuring things are prepared to comfortable down." An early adopter, the store originally advanced hygge as a topic last pre-winter ("we ought to have done it again this year," said Prinsloo). Will hygge last, I asked her? Will it be more than a flash in the plan? "Gracious indeed, certainly. Individuals truly need it and need it right now."

Hygge is catnip to online networking: on Instagram, there are practically 1.5m #hygge posts of falling leaves, bowls of pumpkin soup, and children lovably wrapped in blankets. On Pinterest, there has been a year-on-year ascent of 285% in hygge-themed sticking. Intrigue is particularly strong in Britain, as indicated by a spokeswoman for the site, where "it soar in September this year."

The writer of one of the books on hygge, Meik Wiking, called it "the second Viking attack." In any case, that is not exactly right: hygge has been purposely imported – and reinvented – by enthusiastic Britons. The idea might be permanently Danish, yet the promotion has been made in London. And, amid the clatter and free for all generally 2016, this unexpected preference for shutting the door to the world, for withdrawing back to the hearth, is selling quickly.

Hygge has not shown up in our middle unintentionally. Its presence nearness in Britain involves deliberate inducement and persuasion. In its most clear appearance – the surge of books regarding the matter – it is a pattern that has been deliberately prepared in the lab of London distributing houses, and then scattered through the prepared joint effort of an excited neophile press.

It is book editors – to a great extent youthful, female and brilliant – who made the equation of hygge for a mass British audience. The beginning stage for this youthful way of life chemists was an article that showed up on the BBC site in the main harvest time long stretches of October 2015. Its author, Justin Parkinson, had been throwing around for "news features and zeitgeist articles" from the open-plan breadths of New Broadcasting House, London, four shiny floors over its newsroom. He'd read about hygge in Helen Russell's well-known journal The Year of Living Danishly, and he'd heard the word on a TV cookery program. "I pondered whether I could stir it up into a component," he let me know as of late, so he Googled "hygge UK."

In 2015, the word hygge showed up in 40 pieces in national papers. This year, that figure has shot up to more than 200

"I figured a few people might think it was a slightly poncey, head-scratching thought," he said. Indeed, his article, distributed on 2 October 2015, got over a million hits and was out read that day by just five stories – two pieces on a school shooting in Oregon, and articles on Syria, terrorism, and cancer. It was a little island of cheer on a dismal news day. The article was promptly followed up by others in the Express, the Independent on Sunday, and the Telegraph, the start of a remarkable spike in hygge inclusion: in 2015, the word showed up in 40 pieces in national papers. This year, that figure has shot up to more than 200, a knock of 400% – and that is not including the immense expansion of articles in web journals and way of life magazines.

One individual who saw the BBC article was a distributor named Anna Valentine. She was beginning another engraving, Trapeze, at the publishing aggregate Hachette, whose UK headquarters involve an angular modern building on the north bank of the Thames. The BBC article "ticked such a significant number of boxes on such a large number of levels," she said. Denmark, with its crime show, it is new Nordic cooking, its great plan, its reliable spot at the highest point of national happiness group tables, was "hot," for a beginning. At that point, there was the idea – intriguingly, in a period of Brexit – that "we are seeking different societies for direction on the best way to live our lives. If you take a gander at the greatest selling way of life books, its things like Marie Kondo's The Life-switching Magic of Tidying Up, which is motivated by Japan, at that point, there was Norwegian Wood" – a year ago's non-fiction surprise hit, a Scandinavian tribute to the charms of wood-hacking.

Valentine's point was paradoxical: to distribute books that would be purchased by individuals who "aren't book-purchasers." Hygge appeared to be ideal refining of a famous way of life fixations – starting with care, "which has moved past being a publishing phenomenon and into being a lifestyle, and has taken care of into such a significant number of patterns, as smart dieting books and adult coloring books." She included: "It appeared to integrate with an interest for advanced detox, as well." such a large number of late molds, she stated, had been about self-control and self-hardship – cleaning up, "clean" eating. Hygge "was a cure to all that."

I considered the publishing business offering initial one pattern, and then its cure, as though giving out a succession of uppers and killjoys. The business loves repetitions and hybridizations – crossing one effectively well-known book with another, to concoct another, or new, book, intended to recreate the achievement of previous formulas. (Right now test-tube book-reproducing it is maybe unavoidable that there is a hygge-themed coloring book available this pre-winter. Watch out, as well, for books about lagom – a Swedish word importance lack of abundance – next harvest time.)

Around London, the previous winter, different editors were thinking similar thoughts. In the smooth art deco base camp of Penguin Random House, Emily Robertson and Fiona Crosby were working independently on potential titles for their imprints, Penguin Life, and Michael Joseph. Each had additionally detected the BBC article, they let me know, and when we met in a room of one of the building's echoing marble foyers. "I spend a humiliating measure of my time flicking around the web," said Robertson, "seeing what individuals are reading and sharing on Twitter. Pinterest is large for this. It's an instance of seeing what individuals are discussing."

When the thought had been incubated, the time had come to find writers – yet this was not a clear exercise: the idea of hygge is so underestimated in Danish language and culture that there was no readymade cohort of writers or specialists to approach. The editors needed to either find a willing Dane or recognize somebody with extraneously related information. Valentine reached a specialist she knew, who proposed Charlotte Abrahams, a British author on insides and master on Scandinavian design. Robertson moved toward political specialist Meik Wiking, who runs the Happiness Research Institute, a Copenhagen research organization. Hygge wasn't the sort of thing the establishment looked into, yet the commission was shrewd since the affiliation proposed to the reader that hygge may help provide a shortcut to Danish degrees of prosperity. (The Happiness Research Institute has since become a universal presence in the paper gives an account of the subject, loaning the imprimatur of sociology to the hygge business.) Crosby found Marie Tourell Søderberg, an on-screen character in the Danish authentic dramatization 1864, which had been appeared on BBC4.

For every one of these writers, expounding on hygge was sudden – Wiking disclosed to me his friends were amazed that anybody figured he could get an entire book out of the idea. Abrahams was wanting to compose a book about running; however, she set about assembling a proposition: she had known about hygge, yet not thought about it. (At the point when I visited her at home in the Cotswolds, later, she admitted that candles gave her headaches.)

It was uniquely toward the finish of January, through a partner in the Penguin rights division, that Crosby and Robertson acknowledged they were both publishing books on something very similar. That is despite the way that they work in a similar open-plan office and can see each other from their work areas in case they stand and investigate the heaps of Zadie Smiths and Deborah Levys and Jamie Olivers. The revelation required a meeting over bad coffee, yet it was an amicable experience, not "hygge at sunrise," said Crosby.

So far, Wiking's book has been doing best – a lively exchange at 46,000 copies in the UK, as indicated by Nielsen Book Research, and it is being distributed in 23 different countries. That means that the British, strangely, have become the operators of the dissemination of Danish hygge, as though the general concept had been created in London – which, as it were, it was.

Each book has a diverse flavor. Wiking adopts a broadly sociological strategy, bound with disquisitions on internal design and cooking. Søderberg is a notably pretty book, genial and private, dispersed with reflections from common Danes. Abrahams writes as a foreigner investigating hygge; she consolidates aptitude on Danish structure with a journal ish approach about the quest for satisfaction in her own life.

In any case, for all the sincere social examinations, linguistic glosses and citations from Kierkegaard, it is the pictures, pretty much basic in style to each title that one falls for: hands measuring warm mugs; bikes inclining toward dividers; sheepskin floor coverings tossed over seats; candles and blazes; summer picnics; plate of crisp prepared buns. To see them is to yearn for that life, that glow, that peace, that steadiness – for that idealized, Instagrammable Denmark of the creative mind.

At the point when you show up in Copenhagen, it rapidly turns out to be certain that for Danes, hygge is so inescapable as to be almost invisible. It is utilized in various regular expressions – "Hyg burrow!", or "have hygge," is a typical method for saying goodbye, for instance. It offers itself up flexibly in thing, action word, and adjectival forms, and is a piece of endless mixes: you can tune in to hygge-music, have a hygge-Christmas, and sit in hygge-corner with hygge-lighting maybe appreciating hygge-talk. There is an action word, råhygge, which means, truly, to crude hygge, that is, to appreciate strong, or credible hygge; to hygge with somebody may intend to have a particular sort of sex (and not the surrendered, facing the-cooler kind). As we strolled down a road together in focal Copenhagen, Mette Davidsen-Nielsen, CEO of the paper Information, addressed her telephone to her little girl.

At the point when she completed the concise call, she disclosed to me that she'd utilized the descriptive type of hygge multiple times – "I kept telling her it would be hyggelig to see her."

Hygge's sudden popularity abroad appeared to be both satisfying and bemusing to the majority of the Danes I addressed, as though there was an unexpected fever in Germany for books lauding the deep ideals of British-style saying 'sorry' complete with an exhaustive range of helpful accessories available for procurement. For other people, its break from national limits appeared to be a potential subject of study. "We ought to have a scholastic meeting on the worldwide distinction of hygge," said Carsten Levisen, an associate professor of linguistics at Denmark's Roskilde University. He accepts he is the primary individual to have written a whole scholastic book section on the word from a phonetic point of view. "I amazed myself by having the option to do it," he said.

For all its omnipresence, hygge is additionally perceived as a self-clearly positive and especially Danish worth. Although the word itself is imported from Norwegian, its rise as a component of national culture is some of the time followed back to Denmark's loss of domain in the eighteenth and nineteenth hundreds of years, when it had to abandon tracts of what are currently Norway, Sweden, and Germany. It is sewed further into its language than reciprocals in neighboring countries, (for example, the German Gemütlichkeit, and the Swedish mys) and is firmly entangled with the way that Danish society arranges and extends itself.

You could nearly observe hygge as the private, personal simple of the general population, city Danish government assistance state. Both hygge and the government assistance state depend on a condition of trust, a feeling of smallness (small nation, small circles of friends), and suspicion of equity. Every feed on the other: the government assistance state offers the conditions for hygge to thrive, for it guarantees a 37-hour working week and an opportunity to dedicate to hyggelig exercises; and then again hygge's disdain of hierarchy and conspicuous utilization confers esteems essential to continuing a general public in which distinct contrasts in money related methods are exiled. "In Denmark, our fundamental needs are secured," Marie Tourell Søderberg disclosed to me when she facilitated breakfast for me at her loft – light glimmering, bread directly from the stove. "We don't have to battle for our survival – thus, we have the opportunity to do things that we find important."

Advertisement

Everybody has their own, exceptionally close to the home picture of the most hyggelig hygge. One lively October evening, I got together with a supporter of Søderberg book called Mikkel Vinther, who is an educator of online life at a school that offers proceeding with training to adults. He took me to a Copenhagen public venue. It was facilitating a modest mutual dinner to be trailed by a round of bingo (organized enjoyment is a recognizable component of Danish public activity). There were 200 individuals there; everybody appeared to be youthful, white-collar class, and attractive. Our neighbors at the large public table hung over curiously. "Reason me, are you doing a meeting?" asked one from them. He was called Simon Falk Christensen and filled in as a project manager for Danish State Railways. Interested, he offered his definition. "For me, it's a great deal about the family. Being as one. Candles. It's never about being luxurious, about cakes from the 'right' place. It's a cake you heated yourself. It's a feeling. It's something that has significance in itself, and it is anything but a way to improving as an individual, such as doing exercise. I partner it with being a kid, the smell of my mom cooking onions in the following room. The smell of the Christmas tree."

Over lunch, the next day, Davidsen-Nielsen and her

partner, media observer Lasse Jensen, discussed the importance of hygge. "Intellectualism isn't hygge," said Davidsen-Nielsen. "Extreme discussions on theory and thoughts – that is not very hyggelig. Liquor, sugar, and fat are the three key elements of hygge." He included: "It used to be brew and aquavit, presently its wine." She stated, "There is something in particular about socks and hygge." He included "Hand-knitted socks."

While hygge had numerous varieties, depending on whom you asked, it was constantly hostile to the present day and consistently tinged with nostalgia. Your cell phone isn't hygge. In its local structure, hygge is viewed as basically uncommercial, and by definition, humble, yet simultaneously, it is helped along by certain shopper props – particularly candles or gently glowing lamps.

Davidsen-Nielsen disclosed to me that walking down the road in obscurity, she could investigate her neighbors' windows and spot who was Danish and who was remote, just by their lighting – as though hygge was not only the content of Danishness, yet additionally a sort of social fringe that outcasts couldn't exactly cross. Søderberg, as well, disclosed to me a tale about Syrian outcast friends of hers, who had scanned all over Copenhagen for fluorescent cylinders to light their apartment – the story was told fondly, yet their decision

of residential lighting was a marker of their otherness –
no Dane would settle on a decision so lacking in hygge.
(I had never experienced a comfortable bike shop I
visited Copenhagen – however, their windows were
hung with chic, low-wattage bulbs agleam in the sunset.
Davidsen-Nielsen gave me a fake flame, which is the
coming thing in Denmark, as everybody is beginning to
get stressed over the fact that it is so unhealthy to
breathe candle fumes. It flashes convincingly; it is made
in China.)

To Danes, nothing could be less political than hygge –
since discussing controversial subjects is, by definition,
not hygge – but the idea fits political use. Davidsen-
Nielsen and Jensen disclosed to me that the leader, Lars
Løkke Rasmussen, was hyggelig – the sort of fellow
you could envision enjoying a brew with. "He's folksy
and casual. He's part of the gang. And, he pulls off
homicide – nearly," said Davidsen-Nielsen. "Hygge is
a helpful technique for disguising power. Politically,
you can shroud very forceful or radical acts with an
impression of hygge. Hygge says we should disregard
everything. How about we shut out the world and have
some sweets."

Nothing written on hygge in Britain proposes that it has
a troubling side. Wiking's book mentions that hygge
may, in some cases, feel excluding to outsiders. "It

would be viewed as less hyggelig if there were an excessive number of new individuals at an occasion." Foreigners, he let me know, thinks that it's difficult to enter very close Danish groups of friends: hygge can truly exist inside groups who know each other as of now. Yet, he stops well shy of the investigate that, for example, Dorthe Nors brought to shoulder when we talked. "Incidentally, hygge turned into a type of social control," said the Danish creator, whose novel Mirror, Shoulder, Signal, will be distributed in Britain in February. "It's similar to 'feel-better' in America – the faction of the 'feel-good' book or the 'feel-good' film. It's a cover."

A year ago, Nors distributed a chilling short story, propelled by an article she had found out about a Danish man who had killed his significant other. He was cited as saying, Nors let me know, that he submitted this demonstration not long after the couple had got hyggelig together on the couch. In the story's presentation, she expresses, "Hygge is … utilized as an approach to suppress feelings in a family or relationship. Each time somebody needs to address an unpleasant feeling, this individual is at risk for ruining the hygge and will be told: 'presently, allows just hygge – which fundamentally just methods: Let's remain superficially and carry on hyggelig … It's a wonderful thing, the Danish hygge. And, it's also somewhat risky."

Nors joyfully admitted to a little inconsistency, for she wants to participate in a touch of hygge (she has candles in her office, for instance). Yet, she stated, "You should see us at Christmas. It scares the freak out of me. You're not permitted to be miserable."

The suppression of difference inherent in hygge, Nors stated, was not limited to family life. She related the word to Denmark's truly to a great extent agrarian economy and rustic culture. "its a little country – and we as a whole used to be cultivated, although that is evolving quick. Right now society, conformity is extremely significant. Hygge gives a method for setting up the agreement." Those who cause trouble, who think unexpectedly, who stand up – "they are ruining the hygge," she said.

Besides hygge, there is one other peculiarly Danish thought that guests will in general experience. This is the so-called Jante law – a lot of mentalities said to oversee Danish public activity, depicted in Aksel Sandemose's ironic 1933 novel A Fugitive Crosses His Tracks. The primary principle of the law, which takes its name from the fictional town of Jante, is "You're not to feel that you are anything exceptional," and the others are pretty much a minor departure from that subject: basically, don't get a little too confident. Try not to stick out. Try not to appear as something else.

Sandemose's epic caused debate for its unblinking vision of rural small-mindedness, yet Danes perceive the law of Jante as containing a specific truth: that congruity, and a practically forceful humility, are vital to Danish culture.

These characteristics may advance solidarity and solidarity of a sort valuable in keeping up a libertarian culture, yet it's not hard to see the downsides of social standards that smother singularity or dispute. In the section on hygge in Levison's book Cultural Semantics and Social Cognition: A Case Study on the Danish Universe of Meaning, he describes a tale about Sepp Piontek, the German football administrator who took the Danish national group to their first World Cup in 1986 – and immediately found that hygge was a deterrent to the team's success. "To achieve any outcomes in Denmark, the national group needed to experience a minor social transformation," Piontek wrote in his journal. "The general mentality was that it ought to be fun and hyggelig to be a piece of the national group."

A typical study of hygge, as per Mikkel Vinther, is that it "makes the majority rule process powerless because to talk about difficult things isn't hyggelig." Vinther, himself, is progressively constructive: it has the potential, he contends, to give an amazing, nonconfrontational path for individuals to meet up. But, first, it should be together: he needs to create what he calls hygge 2.0. The way of life services, Bertel Haarder, is setting up a "cultural canon" for Denmark, welcoming Danes to submit thoughts regarding what they generally find significant in their national life. In any case, Haarder himself has sounded a note of alert about setting hygge in such a list – it ought to be done "just if it is something that incorporates instead of, as is regularly the situation, avoids. On apprehensions, I would prefer not to take hygge with us into the future", he said in a meeting not long ago.

Hygge is itself, "where governmental issues are saved," Levisen let me know. In any case, it is this feeling it is past legislative issues – just as its pervasive, final Danishness (and accordingly not-foreignness) – that allows it to be activated by legislators, especially those of the xenophobic far-right, who has become a rising power in Danish governmental issues over the previous decade. (For the individuals who admire Danish society, it came as a disagreeable stun when it was accounted for not long ago that parliament had loved an arrangement to strip displaced people of their resources, including gems and watches, with an obvious unconcern for any disturbing authentic resonances.) An a valid example is Pia Kjærsgaard, the organizer of the counter movement, hostile to Brussels Danish People's

Party, which is, as of now, the second-biggest gathering in parliament. Kjærsgaard has subtly projected herself as the defender of Danish hygge against the obscure powers of the globalized world. As indicated by Nors: "Hygge is a piece of the entire set-up of the extreme conservative in Denmark. Their ads will have all the significant hygge images."

Kjærsgaard, who is currently the speaker in Denmark's parliament, gave a meeting a year ago in which she depicted, in detail, the significance of making her office hyggelig – with family photographs, lights, porcelain, and knickknacks. "I can't flourish and work in workplaces that aren't hyggelig," she said.

Making a hyggelig workplace is normal in Denmark – when I visited the envoy to Britain, Claus Grube, he lit candles, turned off overhead lighting, and put a pad despite my good faith. But, Kjærsgaard and her partners use hygge with specific, and intentional, power, as indicated by Nors, "advancing a famous picture in which being Danish is tied in with sitting cycle a table and eating cake – or pork. Furthermore, they suggest, everybody outside that isn't Danish – and it takes advantage of a dread that globalization and exiles will obliterate everything." The Danish People's Party's point of view is that Denmark is a practically perfect country, with its long history, its liberal government assistance state, and its social distinctiveness. In any case, whatever undermines that safe network, including outsider qualities and philosophies, can't go on without serious consequences.

The softly encoded manner of thinking, at that point, is that if hygge is exceptionally Danish and hygge must be appreciated by insiders, at that point, migrants and outsiders will wreck the country's hyggelig air, and accordingly adequately destroy Denmark. Lotte Folke Kaarsholm, a proofreader on the paper Information, stated, "Obviously hygge prohibits. The entire issue with Scandinavia is that these nations can truly work if you shut the outskirts. You have every one of these standards of consideration within, however for our solidarity to work, you need truly tall walls."

The year wherein hygge has detonated as a British way of life pattern has been extraordinarily turbulent. If 23 June resembled a quake, 8 November was its noting wave – a wonder yet more enormous than the first stun. For each one of the individuals who mourned and worried over the victories of Brexit and Trump, other people celebrated. These unsettling influences uncovered social orders, on the two sides of the Atlantic that is isolated. Youthful versus old, taught versus uneducated, country versus urban, ladies versus men, dark versus white – society's breaks got expanding and self-evident. If years can have temperaments, 2016 was savage in its anger and abject in its fear.

The mind-set of 2016 could even be depicted as u-hygge. The word doesn't, exactly, mean un-cozy – it doesn't gather up sharp-calculated open-plan workplaces with severe furniture. It means frightening; it means sinister. If hygge is sitting round the pit fire, all differences were forgotten, warmed by the moving flames, uhygge is the darkness past that charmed circle. Uhygge, truth be told, takes steps to overwhelm the glow, the solidarity, the consideration. In the unfathomable bleakness of uhygge exist those horrible things from the outside that could destroy you. On some atavistic, profound covered level, transients, displaced people, and those with obviously various qualities carry with them the fearful perfume of u-hygge. In the pressure among hygge and uhygge, the glow of the hearth and the family, and the fear of the lonely world outside, are linguistically bound together. You can see this reflected in Danish culture – most clearly, for those of us in Britain, through its crime drama. Dorthe Nors kidded to me that she thought Nordic noir was a sort of weight release from all the hygge – "all the dim stuff needs to turn out someplace, right?" Watching such projects is a method for keeping uhygge things under control, securely limited in a side of the room, on a screen. The saint of the TV arrangement The Killing, cop Sarah Lund, works in a Denmark that is wet and dark, cold and unforgiving – the chill dark climate and long winters from which hygge is especially skilled at bearing security. She is a long way from the open-air fire. She is distant from everyone else. She is terrible at intimate relationships; she pulls out of rooms where hyggelig family exercises are occurring.

The arrangement, with its darkness and violence, exemplifies uhygge – but then the watcher will, in all probability, experience it from the security and warmth of the family home, a jug of wine open, warming turned up. An analyst story is a method for managing the dark it is tied in with the social events and containing demise and loathsomeness inside a safe and unsurprising account structure. Hygge partners a similar work through various methods: it attracts us towards warmth and togetherness and forgetting. But, it adds some way or another relies upon the presence of the dark, as well. In Wiking's book, there's a comment such that a particularly hyggelig circumstance he recalled (the fragrance of a stew stewing on the stove, an open fire, a group of friends) could have become more hyggelig with the expansion of only a certain something: a raging storm outside.

Hygge is, then, a retreat, an escape, a turning-inwards. If its rise as a component of national culture is regularly followed back to Denmark's loss of domain – a grasp of the personal littleness of recently sharp national borders – maybe its distinctly British symbol masks a comparable national turning-internal, a pulling-up of the drawbridge against the fear of the world.

The editors who urged the British hygge pattern into reality were not weirdly accurate weather forecasters, predicting the full somberness of the conditions to come when they charged their books back in February. In any case, they had placed their fingers in the breeze and, intentionally or something else, found in hygge much that chimed with the times. If this is the year wherein globalization has been found wanting by millions, hygge requests to a prior age, an imagined past, where one could reclaim control or make a nation country once more. The consumerist trappings of hygge, the books and throws and cushions and candles, and holidays and recipes, are not simply sold as items with a specific and practical use, but instead, as mystical articles that may bring up emotions and feelings: of security and comfort, of cozy and quiet, of a being-in-a-period previously. Hygge offers to the two sides of our incredible political partitions: from one perspective, it nostalgically indicates a superior past (of the network, of family, of straightforward delights), and on the other, it offers shelter from the extraordinary, released storms of the occasions.

Carsten Levisen asked as to whether I suspected the craving for hygge in Britain was halfway about a dream of what Britain may have become, f it had gotten the opportunity: Denmark as a sort of option, however, wasted, conceivable future. Maybe, yet if he is correct, it would be a superb logical inconsistency. At the point when Britons are asked whether they need a more grounded government assistance state and greater equity – the nuts and bolts of a more hyggelig life – they will participate in general, vote "no" quite hard. England is ravenous for the accessories of hygge, however not the expenses –, for example, high tax collection – that come with it.

If, for Danes themselves, hygge has a component of imagination – through how it moves once again from challenges, distinction, and discussion – at that point, the British import is a dream of a dream. Hygge might be quintessentially Danish, yet there is something completely British about the nostalgic yearning for the basic accessories of a previous time – particularly if it very well may be purchased. Simultaneously, it is difficult to deny that exactly right now, the most normal thing on the planet is to need to group round the fire and wish the outside away. Settle in: it will be a long winter.

Why individuals are so fixated on 'hygge,'

You may not realize how to articulate it, yet risks are you've felt "hygge" previously.

Request that a Dane clarify the idea, and they'll most likely say hygge is associating with friends and family at home, cuddling in comfortable garments, feeling shielded and safe, getting a charge out of liberal nourishments, drinking reflected on wine and delicate lighting.

"What is particularly Danish is that we have a word that depicts that circumstance," Meik Wiking, a joy analyst situated in Copenhagen, discloses to CNBC Make It. "In any case, there are comparative words the world over that I think catches a portion of very similar things."

Although Wiking didn't develop hygge, his 2017 New York Times top-rated book "The Little Book of Hygge" set hygge up for life and acquainted the Danish solace hypothesis with a worldwide crowd. Google scans for "hygge" in the United States topped that December, as per Google Trends information. On Instagram, individuals began labeling #hygge photographs of heaps of covers on a bed, candles in their home, and cups of steaming cocoa and chunky knit socks. In

March 2018, the Broadway melodic "Frozen" appeared, with a unique tune called "Hygge," with verses like, "Hygge means agreeable, hygge means comfortable, hygge means sitting by the fire with your cheeks all rosy."

There's even a hygge board game sold by Hygge Games that is "intended to start the comfortable discussion." And Nashville-based flame organization Paddywax sells a variety of hygge candles with fragrances like cedar and rosewood. Hygge Life, a retailer that propelled in 2014 in Avon, Colorado, has practical experience in hygge-roused European home merchandise, for example, sheepskin floor coverings and covers. What's more, if that is insufficient, Hygge Box is a membership administration that sends you all that you'd have to hygge for $38 every month.

However, why are individuals so fixated on hygge?

Hygge is something other than a reason to sleep or redesign. Hygge could also be an approach to feel happier during an in any case dark and cold season — something Denmark knows a great deal about.

People today are edgy for anything that gives the vibe great synapse serotonin, similar to kinship, human contact, and embraces, clarifies A. K. Pradeep, a neuro-marketer and creator of "The Buying Brain."

"Strip away the business name of hygge, and what it is at its center is a serotonin sponsor," Dr. Pradeep reveals to CNBC Make It. Throughout the winter months (prime hygge season), individuals around the globe may be longing for exercises that help serotonin and minimize stress.

Wiking says that hygge is "a survival strategy" in Nordic nations, where the winters are long, and it will, in general, get dull around 4 p.m. (However, it very well may be practiced throughout the entire year. "It's hygge to have an outing in the recreation center with your companions or grill," he says.)

Alex Calvert, a geophysicist who moved to Copenhagen from the U.S. nine years prior, reveals to CNBC Make It that he was at first stressed how the hopeless winters and long evenings would influence his temperament.

"In any case, truly, in case you're walking the roads, there's flames and candles in the windows, that are shining with everybody lounging around in covers, having a good visit," he reveals to CNBC Make It. "In this way, even in the depths of winter, there's as yet this feeling of warmth."

According to Dr. Avery, a portion of the principles of hygge, especially socializing, could help somebody coping with the blues. Individuals who are discouraged will, in general, segregate themselves, which escalates their emotions, and leads them to disconnect more; Dr. Avery clarifies. "Associating with friends is significant for any sadness," he includes, "it's critical to associate with individuals."

Hygge social affairs fill in as a smaller than expected custom for individuals to enjoy friendship and "the glow of human organization," Dr. Pradeep says.

Another surprising logical advantage of hygge? Americans will, in general, invest a great deal of energy in PCs or sitting in front of the TV late into the night, which can interfere with their rest, Dr. Avery says.

Hygge, then again, energizes sans screen exercises, for example, reading a book, messing around, or visiting with friends, which could have a more beneficial outcome on your health over the long haul, he includes.

Calvert says that he doesn't have a TV in his family room, yet that hasn't been an issue. Throughout the winter, his hygge routine includes sitting by the fire, reading a book, and having some tea or glass of wine.

(For the record, expending liquor is a hygge health that Dr. Avery wouldn't suggest, particularly for individuals with misery. Liquor meddles with your rest quality, yet additionally can depressive symptoms worse).

A few people, Danes included, accept that hygge does not merit the promotion. Oliver Enné, a 30-year-old imaginative chief who lives in Copenhagen, discloses to CNBC Make It that he doesn't understand "why it's become something like this."

"As a Dane who follows news sources in the U.S., I despise the word hygge," Enné says. "It doesn't mean anything."

The habits regularly connected with hygge, such as spending time with friends or resting by a fire, additionally solid hopeless to Enné. "I think being exhausted with another person is unbearably difficult," he says. "Furthermore, I would prefer to be exhausted all alone than with another person."

Another analysis of hygge, at any rate, how Americans do it, is that there's an excessive amount of focus on hygge items, which detracts from its actual soul. In a 2018 Mashable article, Danish-born essayist Laura Byager expressed: "[A]s soon as hygge is being utilized to sell you stuff you needn't bother with, it loses its importance."

In any case, from a wellbeing point of view, hygge's worth is positive, Dr. Pradeep says. "It's acceptable we're doing it, and it's acceptable we have astute and shrewd approaches to do it," he says. "Nobody should be distraught that some idea from Denmark is being received somewhere else."

Being cozy is good for your health

Snuggle up this season with a warm cover, some tea, and your preferred treat — being comfortable is extraordinary for your well-being. Because of the Danish idea of hygge (articulated hoo-ga), specialists have discovered that embracing comfort and life's little delights can improve by and large satisfaction.

Need confirmation? Danes are viewed as probably the happiest individuals on the planet, as per the 2017 World Happiness Report discharged at the United Nations' International Day of Happiness occasion.

"I consider hygge care enclosed by a sweeping," says Lauren Garvey, MS, CRC, NCC, an instructor and facilitator at Thomas F. Chapman Family Cancer Wellness at Piedmont. "The entire idea is designed for satisfaction, being available, and being agreeable in your body, brain, and space. In our way of life, we are frequently hustling and striving, moving forward at a fast pace. If you are practicing hygge, you are grasping nearness over profitability."

Medical advantages of hygge

Hygge has a wide scope of advantages. It can:

- Increase happiness

- Decrease the adrenal pressure reaction, bringing about fewer cortisol spikes

- Help you be available at the time

- Improve your self-care and self-esteem

- Increase feelings of satisfaction over consumerism

- Combat maladaptive adapting systems, such as spending excessive time on the web or staring at the TV, drinking an excessive amount of liquor or utilizing drugs

HOW TO PRACTICE HYGGE

Here's how to infuse hygge into your life.

- Embrace self-care. Light a few candles and twist up in a comfortable seat with a warm cover, a book or your diary, and a sweet treat if you need one. "Hygge permits us to devote uninterrupted alone time and give ourselves those delights and comforts as a blessing," she says.

- "At the point when we were kids, we frequently had grown-ups soothing us, for example, a parent taking care of us around evening time. You can do that for yourself when you practice self-empathy and self-care."

- Practice self-empathy. "Leave yourself alone. Try not to be no picnic for yourself for not being beneficial at that time or for having a sweet treat," she says.

- Create a cozy environment. "While curating your home, consider the comfort factor," recommends Garvey. "Encircle yourself with whatever is going to assist you with feeling more relaxed and supported." This may mean expelling pointless mess and cleaning up normally, utilizing lights for a comfortable vibe, and choosing agreeable pads and furniture.

- Spend time in nature. Indeed, even in the winter, Danes go for long walks and spend time outside. Investing energy outside has demonstrated pressure mitigating benefits and can assist you with interfacing with an option that is greater than yourself.

- Connect with others. "Social help is a significant part of well-being and health," clarifies Garvey. "Individuals who practice hygge surround themselves with loved ones. It's tied in with interfacing with and appreciating each other's conversation, not contending or impression the board." Spending quality time with others additionally supports feel-great oxytocin, the "cuddle hormone."

- Slow down. If you allow yourself to back off, you'll loosen up your physiology and reduce your adrenal stress responses. "We know from care explore that there are numerous medical advantages to backing off and being available at the time," Garvey says.

- Live at the time. Hygge isn't something you achieve, but instead a way of life. "You don't need to squeeze yourself to do life perfectly," she says. "View life as a journey, not an end state."

173

CHAPTER # 8

CONCLUSION:

At last, offering a dinner or drinks to your friends and family is a key purpose of engaging with hygge. There's no need reason to object about table settings or which fork is right, however. Embrace the simple, easygoing feeling and go for your preferred serving pieces, regardless of whether they're formal or fun. Obviously, wonderful plan can generally be an argument among friends, so don't be hesitant to mention the fanciest piece you possess. For whatever length of time that it brings you and your visitors' satisfaction, nothing is off the menu. Hygge is a decision to back off and enjoy the simple things throughout everyday life. In a world that wears efficient a symbol of respect, hygge is a welcomed respite. Stop the TV, light a flame and wait over supper. Adjust the schedule and set aside a few minutes for appreciation, even in a period of dark and coldness. As we sink into the last a long time of winter, I welcome you go along with me in intentional downshifting. Get those hygge socks on, get yourself a comfortable niche and welcome a portion of your preferred people to go along with you for a treat. While it might be hard to cut out time to enjoy and get comfortable by the fire, basically joining a couple of these practices into your routine can be useful for your well-being. Over and over again we punish ourselves except if we are continually running at most extreme limit, yet it appears to be a few simple joys could be all we have to refuel and prepared ourselves for the stormy days and weeks ahead. With a touch of hygge we also can do as the Danes do, praise reality and change the standard. Although it's easiest demanding to picture hygge in winter, you can surely hygge all year. At the point when the climate is decent, visit your local farmers market and have an outing in the recreation center. Have friends over for a backyard summer barbecue, take the children apple picking, or sit in the shade of a tree and read a decent book. Take a walk on the sea shore, take a dunk in the saltwater, or appreciate a leisurely bicycle ride through town. Take what the season gives you and incline toward it.